Manual of O
Anesthesia 1

M000280856

Fred E. Shapiro, DO
Instructor-in-Anesthesia
Harvard Medical School
Department of Anesthesia, Critical Care and Pain Medicine
Beth Israel Deaconess Medical Center
Boston, Massachusetts

Wolters Kluwer | Lippincott Williams & Wilkins
Health
Philadelphia · Baltimore · New York · London
Buenos Aires · Hong Kong · Sydney · Tokyo

Acquisitions Editor: Brian Brown
Managing Editor: Nicole T. Dernoski
Project Manager: Bridgett Dougherty
Manufacturing Manager: Kathleen Brown
Marketing Manager: Angela Panetta
Design Coordinator: Terry Mallon
Production Service: Laserwords Private Limited, Chennai, India
Printer: RR Donnelley-Crawfordsville

Cover Illustration by Frank D. Fasano, MAMS, BFA

Printed in the USA

Library of Congress Cataloging-in-Publication Data

Manual of office-based anesthesia procedures / [edited by] Fred E. Shapiro.
   p. ; cm.
  Includes bibliographical references and index.
  ISBN-13: 978-0-7817-6908-2
  ISBN-10: 0-7817-6908-6
  1. Anesthesia—Handbooks, manuals, etc. 2. Anesthesiology—Practice—United States—Handbooks, manuals, etc. 3. Anesthesiology—Standards—United States—Handbooks, manuals, etc. 4. Ambulatory surgery. I. Shapiro, Fred E.
  [DNLM: 1. Anesthesia—methods. 2. Ambulatory Surgical Procedures. 3. Anesthesia—standards. 4. Practice Management, Medical. 5. Surgery, Plastic. WO 200 M2947 2007]
  RD82.2.M354 2007
  617.9′6—dc22

                                 2007008651

---

                             10 9 8 7 6 5 4 3 2 1

To my dear sister, Marcelle,
Who taught me a simple life lesson:
Knowledge, determination, and strength
With kindness + health
= achievement with happiness

Contents

Contributors

D. Jonathan Bernardini, MD *Clinical Fellow, Department of Anesthesia, Harvard Medical School, Resident in Anesthesia, Department of Anesthesia, Critical Care, and Pain Medicine, Beth Israel Deaconess Medical Center, Boston, Massachusetts*

Stephanie A. Caterson, MD *Clinical Fellow in Surgery, Department of Surgery, Beth Israel Deaconess Medical Center, Boston, Massachusetts*

Alexander Gerhart *Clinical Resident, Department of Anesthesia, Critical Care, and Pain Medicine, Harvard Medical School, Beth Israel Deaconess Medical Center, Boston, Massachusetts*

E. Cale Hendricks, MD *Chief Resident, Department of Anesthesia, Critical Care, and Pain Medicine, Beth Israel Deaconess Medical Center, Boston, Massachusetts*

Karinne M. Jervis, MD *Clinical Fellow in Anesthesia, Department of Anesthesia, Beth Israel Deaconess Medical Center, Boston, Massachusetts*

M. Jacob Kaczmarski, MD *Clinical Fellow, Department of Anesthesia, Harvard Medical School, Resident in Anesthesiology, Department of Anesthesia, Critical Care, and Pain Medicine, Beth Israel Deaconess Medical Center, Boston, Massachusetts*

Jonathan Kaper, MD *Clinical Fellow in Anesthesia, Department of Anesthesia, Beth Israel Deaconess Medical Center, Boston, Massachusetts*

Kai Matthes, MD *Clinical Resident, Department of Anesthesia, Critical Care, and Pain Medicine, Harvard Medical School, Beth Israel Deaconess Medical Center, Boston, Massachusetts*

Cristin Angley McMurray, MD *Clinical Fellow, Department of Anesthesia, Harvard Medical School, Resident, Department of Anesthesia, Critical Care, and Pain Medicine, Beth Israel Deaconess Medical Center, Boston, Massachusetts*

Jonathon T. Rutkauskas, MD *Department of Anesthesiology, Beth Israel Deaconess Medical Center, Boston, Massachusetts*

Pankaj Kumar Sikka, MD, PhD *Instructor, Department of Anesthesiology, Perioperative and Pain Medicine, Harvard Medical School, Brigham and Women's Hospital, Boston, Massachusetts*

Richard D. Urman, MD *Instructor-in-Anesthesia, Department of Anesthesiology, Perioperative, and Pain Medicine, Harvard Medical School, Attending Anesthesiologist, Department of Anesthesiology, Perioperative, and Pain Medicine, Brigham and Women's Hospital, Boston, Massachusetts*

Preface

This book is the first definitive step-by-step guide to office-based anesthesia. It is intended to have utility primarily for anyone with an interest in this new and burgeoning field, from the anesthesia resident curious about nonhospital practices to the veteran anesthesiologist looking to enter an office-based environment. It also crosses the boundary into various specialties for practitioners who are interested in the office-based setting: e.g., gastrointestinal (GI), ophthalmologists, cosmetic surgeons, dermatologists, oral surgeons, podiatrists, and those who perform interventional cardiac, pulmonary, and neurosurgical procedures. It will delineate, step by step, the creation, maintenance, and optimization of a successful office-based practice, focusing on understanding the entire gamut that comprises the office-based experience.

Chapter 1 outlines what we think are the four key principles of office-based anesthesia: making it *official, safe, pleasant, and comfortable*. It emphasizes the advantages of this novel practice model, the absolute importance of safety measures, and the key steps to combining both into such a practice. *Chapter 2* will outline statistics describing the tremendous recent growth of office-based anesthesia, specifically focusing on the rising popularity of the three most common types of office-based cosmetic procedures: GI, ophthalmology, and cosmetic surgery. In *Chapter 3*, we will examine the members that comprise the office-based perioperative team, specifically delineating the role of the surgeons, anesthesiologists, certified registered nurse anesthetists (CRNAs), and anesthesiology assistants. We also discuss the role of the nonanesthesiologist administering sedation in this setting, specifically who is ultimately responsible for the patient's well-being. The interplay between these parties will be discussed, emphasizing an effective team approach to insure a successful office-based practice. In *Chapter 4*, we will explore the root of the recent growth of office-based anesthesia practice, by answering the question: *Why is office-based anesthesia so popular?* or *What is the allure of an office?*

The office-based setting has been referred to as the "*Wild West of Health Care.*" This is due to a combination of the incentives of decreased cost, convenience, and easy scheduling of cases combined with the exponential growth rate (over the last 10 years) compounded by the fact that currently only 22 out of the 50 states have uniform governmental regulation of the office-based setting on a local, state, or federal level.

With this in mind, *Chapter 5* is a comprehensive in-depth review of all the most current American Society of Anesthesiologists (ASA), American Medical Association (AMA), American College of Surgeons (ACS), regulations and guidelines related to office-based anesthesia, including the ASA patient classification, the definition of monitored anesthesia care (MAC) anesthesia, the delineation of the four different levels of sedation, and the AMA's Ten Core Principles of the Office-Based Practice. A concise in-depth review of these ASA guidelines and recommendations will be made, as a means of providing a uniform standard of anesthesia care to ensure patient safety in a nonhospital setting.

The next section of the manual will provide an in-depth, step-by-step guide to administration of anesthesia in the office.

The first step is to decide whether *the proposed procedure is appropriate to be performed in an office and whether the patient is a good candidate for the procedure to be performed. Chapter 6*, The Preoperative Evaluation, is a concise, comprehensive review of the ASA standards for preoperative care and assessment, patient evaluation, and perioperative testing. It also includes the most current ASA recommendations for preoperative fasting and preparing for drug and dietary supplement interactions with anesthesia.

Chapter 7 answers two important questions: (1) *What are the choices of anesthesia that are available in the office based setting*? and (2) *Which is the safest*? First, we will describe the various anesthetic methods that are most commonly employed in the office. Regional, local, general, and monitored anesthesia care techniques will be discussed, as well as the appropriate patient selection criteria for each type. Second, we will provide an evidence-based in-depth analysis of safety in the office-based setting, utilizing the most current literature that compares the different types of anesthesia and the occurrence and prevention of various operative complications.

To continue the discussion on safety in the office-based setting, *Chapter 8* discusses the ASA closed claims analysis, the most current literature regarding liability during MAC anesthesia, the new use of anesthesia simulation scenarios, and the ASA's closed claims analysis. Established in 1984 as a way to recognize and protect against anesthesia-related complications, the closed claims analysis is one of anesthesiology's greatest tools for increasing patient safety. In the 1990s, the addition and use of the computerized anesthesia simulation was developed as a dynamic means of teaching safety to residents and practitioners with an added incentive for decreasing liability premiums. Currently it is used as an added modality that is incorporated into Accreditation Council for Graduate Medical Education (ACGME) resident teaching programs, for example: *"Calling 911 in the office!"*

These are used as a means of identifying the problems that occur, the types of cases involved, and the mechanism of injury in order to develop safer methods that improve outcomes and standard of care. This is especially prudent in the office-based setting, as the number of reported anesthesia mishaps is limited. The usual time for malpractice claims to be completed and enter the database takes 3 to 5 years, before any change in anesthesia practice can be justified. We often read or hear about the unfortunate high-profile mishaps that occur in the office; however, the latest data dates from 1999 to 2001, lagging 5 years behind. With the doubling of the number of office-based cases over the last 10 years, it would be difficult to calculate an exact number of mishaps or death rates in recent years; the data has yet to be tabulated. *This concise, in-depth, comprehensive manual is a proactive means by which we can address these issues to educate those practitioners involved in the office-based setting to prevent further unfortunate mishaps, perhaps save innocent people while developing a regulated standard of care.*

Chapter 9 will then discuss in detail the preoperative evaluation of the patient, the various anesthetic drugs that are available, and the benefit of the use of various drug combinations. We also review a few issues and controversies regarding the use of "propofol" and discuss the merits of the perioperative use of the newer α_2 agonists. *Chapter 10* is a review of the recommended ASA standards of monitoring, the devices currently available, computerized infusion technology intrinsic to office-based anesthesia, and a few "new" monitors that would be most beneficial for added safety to "sedated" patients undergoing office-based procedures

The next few chapters will examine jointly, from an anesthesia as well as surgical perspective, the most common procedures that are being performed in an office-based setting. *Chapter 11* discusses the *surgical procedures in the office-based setting*. The three most common types are *cosmetic, GI, and ophthalmologic* surgeries. In 2006, 80% of cosmetic surgery was performed in an office or ambulatory surgery center—over 11 million procedures which accounts for billions of dollars. The chapter begins with a description of the seven most common types of cosmetic surgical procedures performed followed by some of the newer, less-invasive nonsurgical cosmetic procedures. The chapter continues with a discussion of oral surgery, podiatric, and interventional cardiac and pulmonary procedures.

We devoted an entire chapter to *ophthalmology* (*Chapter 12*) *and GI procedures* (*Chapter 13*) because these specialties account for a significant number of procedures performed in the office. Each chapter comprises a detailed description of the most common surgical procedures performed and discusses the anesthetic management for each.

Chapter 14 reviews the relatively new area of *Body Contour Surgery* for those patients who experience a significant weight loss either by diet or surgery. We will describe the different procedures that comprise this special subset of surgical procedures, discuss the specific anesthetic considerations inherent in this population, and the significant role that communication plays between the surgeon and anesthesia personnel in order to be safely performed in the nonhospital setting.

To provide a comfortable experience for the office-based surgical patient, *Chapters 15 and 16* are devoted to postoperative pain management. In *Chapter 15*, the traditional methods of pain control are discussed. The various types of anesthetics, the most common drugs, regional blocks as well as the best strategies for use of these are highlighted. These methods are based on the World Health Organization "step-ladder approach" to the treatment of acute postoperative pain in an ambulatory setting. *Chapter 16* provides an evidence-based approach to a few alternative methods to treat acute pain. We describe hypnosis, acupuncture, and music and massage. Each of these can act as an adjuvant to the traditional methods or can be used by itself. We present these complementary approaches to pain management, discuss their plausible mechanisms, and provide evidence to support the merit of employing such techniques in this setting.

We conclude our manual with *Chapter 17*, The Postanesthesia Care Unit, which, for the office-based setting, is probably the most significant. Why? The answer comes from a review from the data that we do have on the ASA closed claims analysis regarding the office-based setting. Of the cases described, the majority could have been prevented by better monitoring, specifically oxygenation through pulse oximetry, in the postoperative period.

We review the most common issues in the postanesthesia care unit (PACU), the differential diagnosis of how to recognize and treat them. We define the Aldrete Score, the criteria for discharge, and the most common causes of unanticipated hospital admissions. We added *appendices* following the PACU chapter that outline the diagnosis and treatment of: (1) *dysrhythmias*, (with the most recent ACLS updates of 2006), (2) *Malignant Hyperthermia* (MHAUS), and (3) the *Difficult Airway* (ASA Task Force 2003). We present the most recent *ASA Guidelines for Office-Based Anesthesia, Ambulatory Anesthesia, and Anesthesia in the Nonoperating Room Setting*.

This is the first comprehensive manual for the practice of anesthesia in the office-based setting. We have provided the most current information, guidelines, procedures, and the choices of anesthesia for this field, which over the last 10 years has grown at an exponential rate. We understand that because of this there are many new issues that arise, which may not be covered in this text. Our ultimate goal is *patient safety*. It is our hope that the use of this manual will educate practitioners, in order to provide a uniform semblance of organization to this Wild West of Healthcare. In doing so, many innocent lives will be saved while a "standard" for the practice of anesthesia in the office and national regulation of this relatively new field is being established.

REFERENCES
1. http://www.plasticsurgery.org/public_education/2006Statistics.cfm.
2. SaRego, M, Watcha MF, White PF. The changing role of monitored anesthesia care in the ambulatory setting. *Anesth Analg*. 1997;85:1020–1036.

3. Lee LA, Domino KB. The Closed Claims Project: Has it influenced anesthetic practice and outcome? *Anesthesiol Clin North Am*. 2002;20(3):485–501.
4. Coldiron B, Shreve E, Balkrishnan R. Patient injuries from surgical procedures performed in Medical Offices: Three years of Florida data. *Dermatol Surg*. 2004;30:1435–1443.
5. Balkrishnan R, Hill A, Feldman SR, et al. Efficacy, safety, and cost of office-based surgery: A multidisciplinary perspective. *Dermatol Surg*. 2003;29:1–6.
6. Vila H, Soto R, Cantor A, et al. Comparative outcomes analysis of procedures performed in physician offices and ambulatory surgery centers. *Arch Surg*. 2002;138:991–995.
7. D'Eramo E, Bookles S, Howard J. Adverse events with outpatient anesthesia in Massachusetts. *J Oral Maxillofac Surg*. 2003;61(983):95.
8. Morell R. OBA questions, problems just now recognized, being defined. *Anesth Patient safety, Found Newsl Spring*. 2000;15:1–3.

Foreword

Office-based anesthesia (OBA) refers to the practice of ambulatory anesthesia in the office setting. OBA is a relatively new and growing field as the number of requests to provide anesthesia services by practitioners who have their own outpatient office-based operating facilities have skyrocketed. Such facilities generally have little regulation at the local, state, or federal level–only 22 of 50 states have any regulations regarding OBA.

The reasons for the tremendous recent growth of interest in this field are many and include the exponential increase in the number of office-based surgical cases performed, the increase in the complexity of these cases, and the increase in the number of patients with major medical problems and risk factors undergoing these procedures. In addition, many of these patients are being sedated by non-anesthesia personnel and there has been an increase in the number of untoward respiratory events reported especially in the postoperative period. Therefore, the tremendous growth of OBA has been accompanied by concerns for patient safety. These concerns have been escalated by media reports of tragedies that may have been precipitated because the physician's office lacked the same resources (i.e., personnel, equipment, drugs, administrative policies and facilities) that are present in an ambulatory surgical center or hospital. In an attempt to maintain quality and safety standards for office-based anesthesia, the American Society of Anesthesiologists (ASA) recently outlined guidelines for an effective system of quality assurance, types of patients suitable for office-based surgery, basic qualifications of office-based surgery personnel, monitoring and equipment standards, and the ability for transfers to hospitals in emergency situations.

This text provides a long-awaited guide to the emerging specialty of office-based anesthesia, filling a need for a reference book in this area. Dr. Shapiro has done a stupendous job composing an easy-to-read yet comprehensive manual which covers all of the idiosyncrasies involved in providing anesthesia to patients in office settings and expounds upon each of the areas noted above. It will provide for the reader a step-by-step practical guide encompassing the entire field of office-based anesthesia

Dr. Shapiro is uniquely qualified to author a text in this field. He has long had an interest in this area and became an innovator in training anesthesia residents in this field when he introduced the first curriculum in office-based anesthesia to the Academy at Harvard Medical School in November of 2005. His manual provides an in-depth comprehensive review of the field and I am confident that this text has all the information necessary to provide practitioners with the skills and knowledge needed to deliver a safe and appropriate anesthetic to patients undergoing surgery in an office-based setting. It will also help familiarize the reader with various aspects of patient care that are often taken for granted in hospital-based operating facilities, such as building code compliance, occupational safety, appropriate patient and case selection, monitoring, equipment maintenance, and emergency protocols. In order to deliver competent care for these patients, a specific knowledge and skills base, that is often inadequately addressed in the traditional anesthesia text, will be covered.

I endorse and support this effort and highly encourage you to read this text whether you are a resident or a practicing physician. In any case it will provide you with a step-by-step up-to-date comprehensive review and guide of this rapidly growing field, as it is in 2007.

Thank you very much.

Carol A. Warfield, MD

Lowenstein Professor of Anesthesia
Harvard Medical School Chairman,
Department of Anesthesia,
Critical Care and Pain Medicine
Beth Israel Deaconess Medical Center

Acknowledgments

There are a number of people to thank whose input over the course of the last 10 years has culminated in the publication of this manual.

In 1997, Dr. Thomas Cochran[1] first initiated me into the world of office-based practice of anesthesia for cosmetic surgery at The Boston Center for Ambulatory Surgery.

It was through this experience that I realized the differences between the office-based and hospital setting. After joining the staff at Beth Israel Deaconess Medical Center Department of Anesthesia Critical Care and Pain Medicine, I, in turn brought this experience to the hospital setting.

It was through Dr. Carol A Warfield's[2] vision and understanding of the added value this has toward improving patient care and resident education that I was afforded the opportunity. She fostered the idea of continuing this practice for which I am most grateful.

Through Dr. Warfield, I was introduced to Dr. Sumner Slavin.[3] It was his motivation that put the wheel in motion for the development of a safer anesthetic practice, especially for aesthetic facial surgery. Through the process of this collegial collaboration he has also become a very dear special friend.

I would like to thank Dr. Stephen A. Cohen[4] for his advice, friendship, and for always being a good listener.

Dr. Peter Panzica[5] for his encouragement, support, and affording me the time to write and edit this manual.

Dr. Donald Morris for supplying photos for the Body Contour chapter, helping to convey that a *picture is often better than words*, and also providing a good game of squash.

Dr. Pedram Aleshi[6] for his research assistance and comprehensive review of the literature.

Tom Steven Xie[7] for his assistance with digital photography and information technology.

Our corporate sponsors Blue Bell Bio-Medical, Nellcor Puritan Bennett (Tyco Healthcare) and OBA-1 (Cardinal Medical Specialties) for their generosity in providing educational grants in support of this project.

Jane Hayward, Hugh Blaisdell, and Tom Laws[8] who could always transform a creative idea into a multidimensional graphic visual display.

Larry Opert, Esq for his wisdom, guidance and legal advice.

Marilyn Riseman for her continued support, encouragement, and friendship.

Finally, my sincere thanks to all the residents who not only assisted with the composition of this manual but also providing the motivation and inspiration behind the development of a *curriculum for teaching safe anesthetic practice in the office based setting*.

[1] Assistant Clinical Professor of Surgery, Harvard Medical School.

[2] Lowenstein Professor of Anesthesia, Harvard Medical School; Chairman, Department of Anesthesia, Critical Care and Pain Medicine, Beth Israel Deaconess Medical Center, Boston, MA.

[3] Clinical Associate Professor of Surgery, Harvard Medical School; Chief, Division of Plastic and Reconstructive Surgery, Beth Israel Deaconess Medical Center, Boston, MA.

[4] Director, Ambulatory Anaesthesia, and Pre-Admission Testing; Assistant Professor of Anesthaesia, Harvard Medical School, Department of Anesthesia, Critical Care, and Pain Medicine, Beth Israel Deaconess Medical Center.

[5] Harvard Medical School; Vice Chairman, Clinical Anesthesia, Department of Anesthesia, Critical Care, and Pain Management, Beth Israel Deaconess Medical Center, Boston, MA.

[6] Resident in Anesthesia Beth Israel Deaconess Medical Center, Boston, MA.

[7] Anesthesia/Clinical Systems Analyst, Department of Anesthesia Critical Care and Pain Medicine, Beth Israel Deaconess Medical Center, Boston, MA.

[8] Media Services at Beth Israel Deaconess Medical Center, Boston, MA.

Principles of Office-Based Anesthesia

E. Cale Hendricks and Fred E. Shapiro

Anesthesia, as a profession and medical specialty, has time and again undergone growth and redefinition. Since the first administration of ether in the 1840s, anesthesiology has grown exponentially. Concurrent with advancements in technology, the field has grown to provide perioperative care to an ever-expanding population, infiltrating virtually every area of modern medical care. Patients with diverse and far-ranging pathology are now routinely carried through invasive and complex surgical procedures. This type of state-of-the-art care has become the expected norm, and it has been possible only with the rigorous drive toward standardized excellence that has marked our profession's growth over the years.

Coexistent with this growth has been change, and, in an admirable way, the practice of anesthesia has evolved to fill each surgical niche virtually as soon as it has appeared. This is especially seen with the advent of cardiac anesthesia in the 1970s and with anesthesia for minimally invasive surgery in the 1990s.

Now a new surgical niche is emerging, and most assuredly our field is evolving to fill it. There are a myriad of ways to state it, but simply put, office-based anesthesia is hot. It is not hard to see why. Office-based anesthesia marries convenience with financial incentive. It is attractive to both surgeon and patient; the former benefiting from greater control over schedule, operating costs, and revenue generation, and the latter gaining in comfort and convenience. One needs look no further than recent national statistics for evidence of the popularity of this emerging subspecialty. In 2005, more than 10 million surgical procedures were performed in doctors' offices. This number has doubled since 1995. Currently, approximately one in ten surgeries are office based (1). This growth has been explosive, and it is sobering when one realizes that in the United States only 22 states currently have legislation regarding office-based surgery. This has led many to characterize office-based anesthesia as the "Wild West" of health care.

This manual is intended to be a survival guide to the office setting. We will provide the current recommendations to a field that is wide open for change. Historically, anesthesiologists have used the closed claims study to improve our practice, using data garnered from past adverse events as a gauge to create a safer anesthetic. There is an inherent problem with this model. It takes 3 to 5 years for the adverse events to come to light, causing an unacceptable delay in the implementation of changes in safer practices. Because the field of office-based anesthesia has grown so rapidly in such a short time, because there exists a lack of regulatory oversight, and because patient safety depends on it, we created this manual to present the latest recommendations to those who need it most.

In the year 2002, the American Society of Anesthesiologists (ASA) published an informational manual titled "Office-Based Anesthesia: Considerations for Anesthesiologists in Setting Up and Maintaining a Safe Office Anesthesia Environment (2)". This manual thoroughly delineates the concerns facing anesthesiologists who are planning on beginning or joining an office-based practice and it gives some very useful guidelines. The advice that is offered is extremely valuable, for it helps the anesthesiologist meet the supreme challenge of office-based anesthesia: to make the care delivered in the office surgical suite tantamount to that delivered in a full-fledged hospital. The specific recommendations from the ASA publication will be presented and elaborated upon later in this text; however, in this chapter we would like to frame the discussion.

Anesthesia in the nonhospital setting is a unique subspecialty with its very own particular challenges and concerns. This book is intended to familiarize the reader with all of these issues and to impart a solid knowledge base to anyone delving into the new field of office-based anesthesia. It is necessary to take a view of this field from the ground up. Focus should first be on the principles underlying office-based anesthesia, which may be summarized by four overarching dictums (see Box 1.1).

Box 1.1

Principles of Office-Based Anesthesia
1. Make it official.
2. Make it pleasant.
3. Make it comfortable.
4. Make it safe.

MAKE IT OFFICIAL

This section should perhaps be titled *Make it "Official"* to reflect the essentially unregulated, unlegislated, nonstandardized current status of office-based anesthesia. Being the relatively new phenomenon that it is, state guidelines for office-based anesthesia have been established in only 22 of 50 states. However, even in the absence of codified regulations, there are certain definite steps that may be taken for making office-based anesthesia practices more official. It should be mentioned here that as the popularity of office-based practices continues to flourish, government and professional organizations should and will increasingly take note. In the near future, full-fledged accreditation and legislation will undoubtedly standardize this new subspecialty. Until this happens, however, the following points will help guide the blossoming formalization of office-based anesthesia.

Accreditation of office-based surgical facilities is currently performed by three organizations (see Box 1.2). Designed to ensure quality care, these organizations lay out definable standards of office-based surgery. In the early 1990s, when rules guiding the practice of office-based anesthesia were truly lacking, an office-based practice would usually only seek accreditation when provoked because of professional competition or for other financial incentives. With the current greater regulatory involvement, however, accreditation is increasingly viewed as a mandate for basic functioning. And as with larger health care organizations, it will eventually become an essential for legal existence.

Box 1.2

• The Joint Commission on Accreditation of Healthcare Organizations (JCAHO)
• The Accreditation Association for Ambulatory Health Care (AAAHC)
• The American Association for Accreditation of Ambulatory Surgery Facilities (AAAASF).

As a surrogate for complete accreditation, the American Medical Association in conjunction with the ASA and the American College of Surgeons recently published a consensus list of principles. Titled the *"AMA Core Principles for Office-Based Surgery"* this list, if not a thorough compilation of every essential for safe office-based surgery, is at best a foundation for safe office-based practice. They may be found in their entirety at http://www.asahq.org/Washington/AMACorePrinciples.pdf and are summarized in Box 1.3.

Box 1.3

1. Guidelines or regulations for office-based surgery should be developed by the states according to levels of anesthesia defined by the ASA.

2. Physicians should select patients for office-based anesthesia by specified criteria including ASA Physical Status Classification System.

3. Where available, offices that perform surgery should be accredited by a state-recognized entity.

4. Physicians involved in office-based surgery should have admitting privileges at a nearby hospital or maintain an emergency transfer agreement with a nearby hospital.

5. Informed consent guidelines should be followed.

6. Continuous quality improvement and adverse incident reporting programs should be kept.

7. All physicians in an office-based setting should be board certified and fully trained.

8. Physicians performing office-based surgery may show competency by maintaining privileges at an accredited hospital or ambulatory surgical center for the procedures they perform in an office setting.

9. At least one physician who is credentialed in advanced resuscitative techniques (advanced trauma life support [ATLS], advanced cardiac life support [ACLS], or pediatric advanced life support [PALS]) must be present or immediately available with appropriate resuscitative equipment until the patient has met discharge criteria.

10. Physicians administering or supervising the anesthetic should have appropriate education and training.

Finally, professional liability coverage is an essential that must be considered carefully. Just as anesthesia is evolving to fill the office niche, insurers are likewise in the process of evolution. The same coverages that have worked for the anesthesiologist in the hospital setting will not necessarily translate to the office setting. It is extremely important that the office-based anesthesiologist be familiar with his or her professional liability policy including its declarations, amendments, attachments, and qualifications.

MAKE IT PLEASANT

The next dictum for establishing a good office-based anesthesia practice is to make the entire office-based perioperative experience a pleasant one. The ability to reinvent the traditional surgical experience is one of the most important reasons behind the emergence of anesthesia in the office setting.

To contrast with many hospital experiences, a good office practice should be relaxing, comfortable, and convenient for all involved. For the patient this involves ease of arriving to the office surgical suite. It also means ease of passage through a surgical experience that occurs in a comfortable, non-threatening atmosphere. This may be accomplished simply by well-mannered staff and a relaxing preoperative area, or it may be accomplished by ushering the patient from a living room–like holding area to an operating room (OR) adorned with art to a softly lit and aesthetically pleasing postanesthesia care unit (PACU). Advances in analgesic drugs and a growing awareness of complementary techniques, in the hands of skilled personnel, can help ease a patient smoothly into postsurgical recovery. The aim should be a pleasing experience for the patient, family, and friends. The end result may, in fact, be a Zen-like atmosphere with quiet music and soft speech—likened to a spalike experience.

MAKE IT COMFORTABLE

The anesthesiologist plays an integral role in helping to make the perioperative experience pleasant for the patient. More than that, however, the anesthesiologist can *benefit* from a well-conceived, well-structured office environment. In contrast to the ordinary procedure room, the ideal office operating suite will have a spacious, ergonomically designed OR. Monitors should be easily viewable, chairs should be comfortable, and anesthesia equipment should be modern and in good repair. Methods for obtaining, storing, and dispensing medications should be straightforward and hassle free. Holding area, operating suites, and PACUs should be contiguously located to allow for seamless flow of transport. One would not want to walk into an office, regardless of the financial incentive, if the equipment and infrastructure is antiquated, cumbersome, or ill functioning. Building an effectively functioning office-based practice can be a very challenging business, but when properly executed, the office-based environment can be the ideal place of work for an anesthesiologist.

MAKE IT SAFE

The safety of the patient is the foremost obligation of the anesthesiologist in any setting. This tenet should remain steadfast regardless of the location of the surgical procedure; from acute-care hospital to office-based facility, all anesthesia safety standards must be maintained. Safety features that are taken for granted or even unnoticed in an acute care hospital must be carefully built into a new office operating suite or retrofitted into an existing one.

- *Fire safety* must be considered. The office building must be easily evacuated if such need arises. There must be a sizable enough workspace to easily accommodate patient, bed, OR table, equipment, and personnel and still leave plenty of room for maneuvering. It is critical that in multistory buildings this includes elevators of sufficient size to transport a ventilated patient in a stretcher with monitors and associated care providers.
- A tenable *emergency transportation* plan should be in place and ready for action should the need arise. This should include rapid and efficient transfer to a hospital equipped to provide a higher level of care in critical situations.
- *Air handling* is another concern, as adequate ventilation, air-conditioning, and heating must be available for individual ORs.
- *Electrical systems* must have independent sources of alternate power in the event of primary electrical service interruption. To conform to National Fire Protection Association guidelines for health care facilities, alternate power must, at the minimum, be effective for 1.5 hours, providing enough light and power for life safety and the orderly termination of a procedure.

Setup, maintenance, and administration of *medical gases* introduce another limb of safety that is of critical importance for the delivery of any anesthetic.

- *Oxygen* must be available whether distributed from a central source (preferred) or through portable tanks. If tanks of compressed gas are to be used, they must be routinely inventoried, transported, and stored safely.
- *Vacuum* sources must be available with backup in the event of power failure.
- *Gas scavenging systems* must be employed for any planned administration of potent inhalational agent or nitrous oxide.

Also, in the office setting, provisions must be made to accomplish tasks usually carried out by hospital-based ancillary staff. Equipment must be disinfected and/or sterilized, procedure rooms must be cleaned, and biohazardous waste and sharps must be properly disposed of. Before the anesthesiologist even steps into the office-based operating suite, much infrastructure must be in place to provide a foundation for the delivery of a safe anesthetic.

It must be remembered, however, that this is merely the foundation. It takes the entire perioperative team (rigorously observing all accepted perioperative standards of care) orchestrating their efforts to ensure the uncompromised delivery of safety in the office environment. By being a bit creative, by thinking outside of the box, we can stay ahead of the game. We can keep up with the trends in health care, we can protect ourselves from unsafe working conditions, and, most importantly, we can protect our patients from being a statistic. When all things are considered, patient safety should always come first.

REFERENCES

1. American Society of Anesthesiologists. *Office-based anesthesia and surgery.* http://www.asahq.org/patientEducation/officebased.htm. Last accessed November 2006.
2. ASA Task Force on Office-Based Anesthesia. *Considerations for anesthesiologists in setting up and maintaining a safe office anesthesia environment.* http://www.asahq.org/publicationsAndServices/office.pdf. Last accessed November 2006. 10 May 2002.

The Statistics

Jonathon Rutkauskas and Fred E. Shapiro

Provision of surgical services on an outpatient basis and particularly in an office-based setting has risen dramatically during the last decade. According to the American Society of Anesthesiologists (ASA), an estimated 10 million procedures were performed in doctors' offices in 2005—twice the number of office-based surgeries performed in 1995 (see Figure 2.1). The trend toward office-based surgery parallels the growing trend ambulatory surgery experienced a few years ago, and now approximately one in ten surgeries are performed in physicians' offices (1). This correlates with a strong need for competent anesthesiology personnel to perform services in office-based settings. But what types of procedures are being performed in physicians' offices?

Most procedures that can be performed on an outpatient basis can also be performed in a physician's office. Unfortunately, no adequate data collection exists to pinpoint exactly how many office-based surgeries are performed, a number that shifts depending on how one defines office surgery. A list of the more common outpatient procedures, all of which are also commonly performed in physician's offices, can be found in Box 2.1.

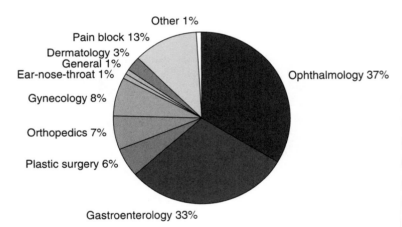

Figure 2.1. Office-based procedures. (Source: Based upon 2003 Medicare Data Federation for Ambulatory Surgery in America.)

Box 2.1

Surgical specialties that perform most office-based procedures include *gastroenterology, ophthalmology, plastic surgery,* dentistry, podiatry, gynecology, otolaryngology, orthopedics, and general surgery.

Table 2.1. Most common outpatient procedures, 2004

Name	Volume
Colonoscopy	239,630
Extracapsular cataract removal with insertion of IOL technique	208,352
Upper gastrointestinal endoscopy *with biopsy*	176,940
Colonoscopy *with removal of tumors, polyps, or other lesions*	90,944
Injection of *diagnostic or therapeutic substances* epidural or subarachnoid; lumbar, sacral	90,862
Colonoscopy *with biopsy—single or multiple*	87,092
Lens; laser surgery	68,553
Colonoscopy *with removal of tumors, polyps, or other lesions by electrocautery*	66,505
Fetal nonstress test	49,396
Debridement; skin and subcutaneous tissue	41,604
Transfusion—blood or blood components	36,601
Introduction/injection of *anesthetic agent,* diagnostic or therapeutic, lumbar or sacral, single level	34,531
Upper gastrointestinal *endoscopy*	34,134
Arthroscopy of the knee; with meniscectomy	29,071
Spinal injection	23,026

IOL, intraocular lens.
Source: This information is from "FHA Eye on the Market: Outpatient surgery report, September 2005," which includes data on individual hospitals.

Table 2.1 shows a breakdown of the top 15 outpatient procedures in their various subspecialties, all of which can be performed in physician's offices. The areas *highlighted* denote the differences between similar types of listed procedures.

Particularly prevalent in regard to the office-based setting is the exponential increase in the number of procedures performed by plastic surgeons. The American Society for Aesthetic Plastic Surgery (ASAPS) releases yearly statistics from its data bank showing yearly trends as well as the most popular procedures. According to the most recent statistics released by ASAPS there were approximately 11.5 million surgical and nonsurgical cosmetic procedures performed in the United States in 2005. Since 1997 there has been an increase of 444% in the total number of procedures, a trend which can be viewed in Figure 2.2.

Boxes 2.2 and 2.3 list the top five surgical and nonsurgical cosmetic procedures. Table 2.2 lists the number of these procedures performed in 2005.

Box 2.2

According to the ASAPS data for all Americans in 2005, the top five *surgical* cosmetic procedures were *liposuction, breast augmentation, eyelid surgery, rhinoplasty,* and *abdominoplasty.*

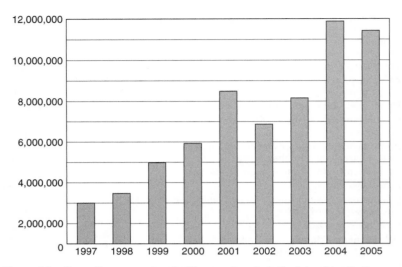

Figure 2.2.   Cosmetic surgery trends. (Source: American Society of Aesthetic Plastic Surgery.)

Table 2.2.   Top surgical and nonsurgical cosmetic procedures among all Americans in 2005

Surgical	No. of Procedures	Nonsurgical	No. of Procedures
Liposuction	455,489	Botox	3,294,782
Breast augmen-tation	364,610	Laser hair removal	1,566,909
Eyelid surgery	231,467	Hyaluronic acid treatment	1,194,222
Rhinoplasty	200,924	Microdermabrasion	1,023,931
Abdominoplasty	169,314	Chemical peel	556,172

Table 2.3.   Top five cosmetic surgeries for women in 2005

Liposuction	402,946
Breast augmentation	364,610
Eyelid surgery	198,099
Tummy tuck	164,073
Breast reduction	160,531

Table 2.4.   Top five cosmetic surgeries for men in 2005

Liposuction	52,543
Rhinoplasty	45,945
Eyelid surgery	33,369
Male breast reduction	17,730
Face-lift	13,041

Box 2.3

The top five nonsurgical procedures were *Botox, laser hair removal, hyaluronic acid treatments, microdermabrasion*, and *chemical peel*.

Tables 2.3 and 2.4 show the variation in cosmetic procedures performed on women and men. According to ASAPS, despite the 15% decrease in the number of surgical procedures in men from 2004 to 2005, the total number of cosmetic procedures, both surgical and nonsurgical, performed on men has increased 306% from 1997 to 2004. This exponential increase can be attributed to men's growing interest in nonsurgical procedures (see Boxes 2.4 and 2.5).

Box 2.4

Women comprised *91.4%* of the total cosmetic procedures = 10.5 million (decrease of 2% from 2004).
Men had approximately *9%* of the total cosmetic procedures = 985,000 (15% decrease from 2004) (3).

Box 2.5

The Distribution of the Percentage of Cosmetic Surgeries by Age-group
Younger than 18 = 1.5% of procedures
19 – 34 = 24%,
35 – 50 = 47%(5.3 million = most procedures)
51 – 64 = 24%
Older than 65 = 5%

With roughly three out of every four cosmetic surgical procedures being performed in an office or surgicenter, it is prudent for anesthesiologists to be prepared for the specific issues that are unique to the office setting (see Box 2.6).

Box 2.6

In 2005

48% of cosmetic procedures were performed in an office facility.
28% of procedures were performed in a freestanding surgicenter.
24% of procedures were performed in a hospital.

The high volume of cosmetic procedures, particularly those being performed in an office, is overshadowed only by the inordinate rate of growth that has occurred over the last 10 years. On this basis, it is crucial for anesthesiology personnel to provide services in a safe, effective manner commensurate with the ease, convenience, and cost incentives presented by the office-based setting. If one evaluates the trends, it appears that over the next few years there will be an even greater demand to accommodate such an impressive surgical volume.

REFERENCES
1. American Society of Anesthesiologists. *Office based anesthesia and surgery.* American Society of Anesthesiologists; Last viewed 11/16/06. http://www. asahq.org/patientEducation/officebased.htm. 2006.
2. FHA Eye on the Market. *Outpatient surgery report.* Sept. 2005.
3. American Society of Aesthetic Plastic Surgery. *Cosmetic surgery national databank.* 2005.

Members of the Team

Jonathon Rutkauskas and Fred E. Shapiro

When considering safety in office-based anesthesia one must recognize that both the surgery and the anesthesiology personnel should act as a "team". The surgical procedure entails a coordinated effort, as the surgeon operates while the anesthesiology care team maintains constant "vigilance" to adhere to a safe anesthetic plan. This chapter will devote attention to the physicians performing the procedures and the anesthesia personnel, both of whom comprise the "members of the team".

As discussed in Chapter 2, office-based surgical procedures encompass a wide array of medical specialties. The physicians who are most prevalent in the office-based setting are listed in Box 3.1. Each of these specialties holds its own training requirements and certification process to ensure that its members have achieved appropriate expertise in their fields. The scope of this chapter is not to discuss every subspecialty and their respective qualifications, more so to convey the message that *the same standards and qualifications should prevail whether the practice is in an office or a hospital*.

Box 3.1

Physicians Most Prevalent in Office-Based Practice
Plastic surgeons
Gastroenterologists
Oral surgeons

Otolaryngologists
Podiatrists
Ophthalmologists

Plastic surgeons, for example, often operate in office-based settings. In order to be board certified, one must complete at least 5 years of residency after medical school. He or she must then pass comprehensive written and oral exams in order to become a diplomate of the American Board of Plastic Surgery. Those plastic surgeons who wish to focus exclusively on cosmetic procedures must pursue the additional training necessary to attain membership in the American Society for Aesthetic Plastic Surgery (ASAPS) (1).

The anesthesia care team maintains an equally important role in determining the success of an office-based surgical practice. Anesthesia care teams are led by anesthesiologists who directly provide patient care or delegate responsibility to appropriate members of the team. Members of the anesthesia care team who also assist in providing direct patient care during the perioperative period include anesthesiologists certified registered nurse anesthetists (CRNAs), and anesthesiology assistants. The common denominator amongst anesthesia personnel is that they are highly trained in airway management and have the ability to deal with all perioperative emergencies. See Box 3.2 for a more detailed description of each member of the team.

Box 3.2

Members of the Anesthesia Care Team

1. *Anesthesiologist:* MD or DO who has completed an accredited (minimum of 4 y) residency program after 4 y of medical school. In order to be board certified, one must also pass both a comprehensive written and oral exam.

2. *CRNA:* RN who has completed a 4-y degree, followed by 1- to 2-y experience in acute care nursing, followed by 2–3 y of accredited CRNA education, then passed national certification exam.

3. *Anesthesiology Assistants (AA):* Bachelor's degree, followed by 2.5 y in an AA-accredited program, then passed national certification exam—AAs have duties and safety rates equivalent to CRNAs.

Regardless of who is providing direct anesthetic care, the American Society of Anesthesiologists (ASA) policy documents that all anesthetics *should* be delivered by or under the medical direction of an anesthesiologist, and that anesthesiologist participation in office-based surgery is optimally desirable as an important patient safety standard (2). The ASA maintains separate guidelines concerning the administration of conscious sedation by the nonanesthesiologist, requiring formal training in the use of anesthetic drugs that provide moderate sedation and the ability to rescue patients who exhibit deeper-than-intended levels of sedation (3).

Surgeons and anesthesiologists both endure years of rigorous training with the common goal of providing optimal care for their patients. The office-based setting emphasizes how crucial it is for physicians to utilize the 'team approach' in order to provide each patient with the safest, most pleasant, and comfortable experience.

REFERENCES

1. The American Society of Aesthetic Plastic Surgery. www.surgery.org. 2005.
2. American Society of Anesthesiologists. *Office-based anesthesia and surgery*. http://www.asahq.org/patientEducation/officebased.htm. Last accessed November 2006.
3. American Society of Anesthesiologists Task Force on Sedation and Analgesia by Non-Anesthesiologists. Practice guidelines for sedation and analgesia by non-anesthesiologists. *Anesthesiology*. 2002;96:1004–1017. http://www.asahq.org/publicationsAndServices/sedation1017.pdf (last accessed November 2006.)

The Allure of an Office

Jonathon Rutkauskas and Fred E. Shapiro

Over the last 20 years there has been an impressive shift in numbers from inpatient to outpatient surgery. Upon questioning, most people would prefer to enjoy the comforts of their own home and not be admitted to the hospital postoperatively. This is only one of the reasons ambulatory surgery has attained such popularity. Newer less invasive procedures, shorter acting medications, and computer-assisted technology have also helped propel an "in and out" the same day procedural philosophy. Approximately 80% of all surgeries are currently performed in outpatient facilities, either connected to hospitals or in separate surgical centers (1). More recently there has been a rising trend for surgery to be performed within the physician's office (see Figure 4.1).

Office-based surgery can offer the convenience of having procedures performed in a more comfortable setting with an expedient return home (1). To entice and titillate the consumer, doctors' offices have been furnished with modern art, classical antiques, Zen-like minimalist Feng Shui design, scented candles, water fountains, soothing music, cashmere blankets, and even wheat germ smoothies of assorted green and white anti-oxidant teas—just a few of those "spalike touches" that appeal to the senses.

The American Society of Anesthesiologists (ASA) reports that in 2005 an estimated 10 million procedures were performed in physicians' offices, twice the number of office-based procedures performed in 1995 (1). In addition to the aesthetics described in the preceding text, office-based surgery provides flexibility and ease of scheduling, as well as increased efficiency compared with hospital-based surgery.

Because numerous types of surgical procedures are being performed, a wide range of anesthetic techniques are also available. The continuum of these ranges from light sedation or anxiolysis to general anesthesia. Providing services in an office-based setting is a prime opportunity for anesthesiologists to practice in an environment slightly different than the traditional hospital setting. The office setting presents its own unique challenges. It emphasizes the importance of the anesthesia personnel's role as true perioperative physicians, those who are present throughout the 'pre-, intra-, and postoperative period'.

In addition, it is also an environment that requires a more social interaction in order to appease, support, and nurture the patient. It is a time for anesthesiologists to showcase their personalities to enhance the patient's feeling of importance and self esteem while still delivering safe anesthetic care.

The office-based setting is discreet, nurturing, and hassle free, so why is it often termed the "Wild, wild west" of health care?

One major fundamental difference between office-based facilities and hospitals or surgicenters is that the strict, well-defined standards and regulations that maintain safety both in surgery and anesthesia that are in place in hospitals and surgicenters do not uniformly apply to physicians' offices in the United States (1). Currently, only *22 states* require the same standards in doctors' offices as they do in hospitals and surgicenters (2). The number of office-based surgical facilities that are actually accredited, licensed, or certified is limited not because they are deemed substandard, but rather because there is no current uniform mandate that regulates the office-based setting nationally.

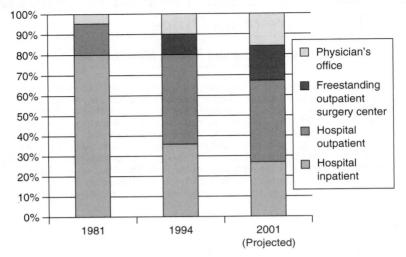

Figure 4.1.   Location/setting of anesthesia procedures (by percentage). Location of anesthesia procedures. (Twersky RS. The anesthesiologist in the ambulatory care setting. *ASA Newsl.* **1996;60:11–13.)**

Published data has shown that the office-based surgical facilities that are accredited have a safety record comparable to that of hospital ambulatory surgery settings (see Chapter 7).

Is there a governing body that confers accreditation status upon these centers? Office-based surgical facilities can be accredited by a nationally or state recognized agency, or can be state licensed or medicare certified. Specific nationally recognized accreditation agencies are listed in Box 4.1 (3).

Box 4.1

American Association for Accreditation of Ambulatory Surgery Facilities **(AAAASF)**

The Joint Commission on Accreditation for Healthcare Organizations **(JCAHO)**

The Accreditation Association for Ambulatory Healthcare **(AAAHC)**

These agencies regularly inspect such offices ensuring that minimum standards of patient care are met.

The fact that mandatory standards and regulations are limited does not mean that the medical community is ignoring patient needs. In fact, both the American Society of Aesthetic Plastic Surgery (ASAPS) and the ASA express commitment to ensuring patient safety in their mission statements (4). Both societies urge prospective patients to make sure that their office-based surgery meets certain requirements. As of July 2002, in support of this, all ASAPS members have agreed to perform cosmetic procedures which require anesthesia only in accredited, state licensed, or medicare-certified facilities. In addition to board certification, the ASAPS promotes the recommendations listed in Box 4.2.

Box 4.2

Recommendations for Safety in Office-Based Surgery by the ASAPS

1. The office-based facility is nationally accredited or state licensed.
2. The surgeon has privileges at an acute care hospital for the specific procedure being performed.
3. The emergency equipment and anesthetic monitoring devices should be equivalent to those in a hospital or surgicenter (including emergency drugs and equipment to handle rare life-threatening complications).
4. Provisions are available for hospital admission if unforeseen complications arise.
5. There is a separate recovery area equivalent to a hospital or surgicenter.
6. Until the patient is fully recovered, a physician and an RN are at the site.

The *ASA* is also intricately involved in contributing to policies for office-based anesthesia. In conjunction with the *American Medical Association* (*AMA*) and the *American College of Surgeons* (*ACS*), the ASA was instrumental in constructing the *AMA Core Principles on Office-Based Surgery*—a document endorsed by more than 35 organizations at a consensus conference and last updated in 2005 (5). Initially approved in 1999, the ASA has also approved its own set of guidelines for office-based anesthesia that focuses on patient safety and anesthesia quality. The ASA further states that the existing guidelines for ambulatory anesthesia should be followed because office-based anesthesia is considered a subset of ambulatory anesthesia (4). In the next chapter, these specific guidelines created by the ASA will be outlined and reviewed.

In the properly accredited office setting the overall goal of anesthesia and surgery is to provide a safe, pleasant, and comfortable experience for the patient. This environment offers the anesthesiologist its own challenges coupled with a different "style" of practice. It is prudent to develop the skills of "a true perioperative physician", an anesthesiologist who is present throughout the pre-, intra-, and postoperative period. What makes the office-based setting most unique? It is here that the primary role of the physician as both the "caregiver and nurturer" is commonly combined.

REFERENCES

1. American Society of Anesthesiologists. *Office-based anesthesiology and surgery*. American Society of Anesthesiologists; www.asahq.org/patientEducation/officebased.htm. (Last accessed November 2006). 2001.
2. Anesthesiology Info. *Office-based anesthesia: new standards needed for anesthesiologists*. www.anesthesiologyinfo.com/articles/01092002b.php. (Last accessed November 2006). Posted May 3, 2000.
3. American Society for Aesthetic Plastic Surgery. *Office surgery: guidelines for patient safety*. http://www.surgery.org/press/news-release.php?iid=148&section=news-credentials (Last accessed November 2006). February 27, 2004.
4. American Society of Anesthesiologists. *ASA guidelines for ambulatory anesthesia and surgery*. http://www.asahq.org/publicationsAndServices/standards/04.pdf. (Last accessed November 2006). October 15, 2003.
5. American Medical Association. *Improving office-based surgery*. http://www.ama-assn.org/ama/pub/category/11807.html. (Last accessed November 2006). August 10, 2005.

American Society of Anesthesiologists' Guidelines for Office-Based Anesthesia Practices

Richard D. Urman

In this section, some key regulations and guidelines related to the office-based anesthesia (OBA) practice are reviewed. Over the last 10 years, a large increase in office-based procedures has forced the American Society of Anesthesiologists (ASA) and other professional societies to come up with specific guidelines to promote patient safety and professional quality. Most of the information can be found in the ASA literature, and much of the detailed, current information is available on the ASA website (www.asahq.org). Unfortunately, there is still limited regulation of the office-based facilities in most states, and most federal and state laws do not go far enough (1).

The ASA encourages the anesthesiologist to play a leadership role as a perioperative physician in all hospitals, ambulatory surgical centers, and office-based settings. The guidelines and recommendations discussed in the subsequent text apply to anesthesiology personnel administering ambulatory anesthesia in all settings. Most are minimal basic guidelines, which may be exceeded at any time based on the judgment of the involved anesthesia personnel. It is also noted that these guidelines encourage high-quality patient care, but by observing them one cannot guarantee any specific patient outcome. One of the recent positive developments came in July 2002, when all American Society for Aesthetic Plastic Surgery (ASAPS) members agreed to perform surgeries that require anesthesia (other than local anesthesia and/or minimal oral or intramuscular tranquilization) only in an accredited, state-licensed, or Medicare-certified facility. The ASA believes that when proper guidelines are followed, office-based surgery is a safe, convenient, and cost-effective option for properly selected patients.

One of the most thorough documents recently published by the ASA is an information manual assembled by the ASA Committee on Ambulatory Surgical Care and the ASA Task Force on Office-Based Anesthesia (2). This work, titled *Office-Based Anesthesia: Considerations for Anesthesiologists in Setting Up and Maintaining a Safe Office Anesthesia Environment,* is available on the ASA website. Its authors wanted to "expand on the recommendations of the ASA guidelines for office-based anesthesia," and provide "advice and resources for anesthesiologists who currently practice, or plan to practice, in the office setting." This document discusses various topics critical to maintaining a safe office-based practice, such as facility accreditation; provider credentials and qualifications; principles of facility safety, medication management, preoperative, intraoperative, and postoperative care; and monitoring and equipment. It also discusses the management of emergencies.

While it is impossible to cover all aspects of OBA-related rules and guidelines in this chapter, it is important to mention a few major developments in this area. Box 5.1 shows the list of recent ASA documents that are relevant to the anesthesia practice in an office setting (see Appendix 1).

Box 5.1

1. **Guidelines for Office-Based Anesthesia**
2. **Guidelines for Ambulatory Anesthesia and Surgery**
3. **Statement on Qualifications of Anesthesia Providers in the Office-Based Setting**
4. **Guidelines for Nonoperating Room Anesthetizing Locations**
5. **Position on Monitored Anesthesia Care**
6. **Office-Based Anesthesia: Considerations for Anesthesiologists in Setting Up and Maintaining a Safe Office Anesthesia Environment (ASA Committee on Ambulatory Surgical Care and ASA Task Force on Office-Based Anesthesia)**
7. **Statement on the Anesthesia Care Team**
8. **Practice Guidelines for Sedation and Analgesia by Non-Anesthesiologists**
9. **Standards for Basic Anesthetic Monitoring**
10. **Continuum of Depth of Sedation Definitions of General Anesthesia and Levels of Sedation/Analgesia**
11. **Standards for Post-Anesthesia Care**
12. **Guidelines for Determining Anesthesia Machine Obsolescence**

The *ASA Guidelines for Office-Based Anesthesia* were first approved by the ASA House of Delegates in 1999, and reaffirmed in 2004. It was primarily intended for anesthesiologists practicing ambulatory anesthesia in office-based environments (1). The ASA recognizes the unique needs of an OBA setting and the increased requests for ASA members to provide anesthesia for health care practitioners (physicians, dentists, podiatrists) in their office-based operating rooms. The ASA states that because OBA is a subset of ambulatory anesthesia, the ASA guidelines for ambulatory anesthesia should be followed in the office-based setting as well as the ASA standards and guidelines that are applicable.

The ASA also recognizes the fact that compared with acute care hospitals and licensed ambulatory surgical facilities, office suites have limited, if any, regulation or control by federal, state, or local laws. Therefore, the onus is on the anesthesiologist to satisfactorily investigate areas taken for granted in the hospital or ambulatory surgical facilities, such as governance, organizations, construction, and equipment, as well as policies and procedures, including fire, safety, drugs, emergencies, staffing, training, and unanticipated patient transfers. The anesthesiologist is encouraged to address those issues in an office setting before administering anesthesia. It involves the personnel, facility, administration, and developing a plan for the pre-, intra-, and postoperative care of the patient. Because of the rapidly growing numbers of procedures being performed in the office-based setting, further recommendations were approved by the House of Delegates in 2004. These involve the quality of care and patient safety in the office setting.

The Guidelines for Office-Based Anesthesia address six major aspects of office-based practice.

1. *Quality of care*
2. *Facility and safety*
3. *Patient and procedure selection*
4. *Perioperative care*
5. *Monitoring and equipment*
6. *Emergencies and transfers*

It is important to consider each of the topics listed in the preceding text in detail, because each is critical to a safe, effective, and quality anesthetic. This chapter will address each aspect of the guidelines separately, and discuss other relevant literature, regulations, and recommendations.

QUALITY OF CARE

The Guidelines for Office-Based Anesthesia first address the administration and facility aspects of the office-based practice (see Box 5.2). They call for the facility to have established policies and procedures that are to be reviewed on an annual basis. Such a facility would need to have a governing body and/or a medical director who supervises the staff and ensures that appropriate procedures are being performed and that the personnel are properly trained. It calls for properly licensed and educated practitioners, and for the anesthesiologist to partake in continuing education, quality improvement, and risk management activities.

Box 5.2

The Guidelines for Office-Based Anesthesia Based on Facility and Administration

- The facility should have a medical director or governing body that establishes policy and is responsible for the activities of the facility and its staff.
- The medical director or governing body is responsible for ensuring that facilities and personnel are adequate and appropriate for the type of procedures performed.
- Policies and procedures should be written for the orderly conduct of the facility and reviewed on an annual basis.
- The medical director or governing body should ensure that all applicable local, state, and federal regulations are observed.
- All health care practitioners[1] and nurses should hold a valid license or certificate to perform their assigned duties.
- All operating room personnel who provide clinical care in the office should be qualified to perform services commensurate with appropriate levels of education, training, and experience.
- The anesthesiologist should participate in ongoing continuous quality improvement and risk management activities.
- The medical director or governing body should recognize the basic human rights of its patients, and a written document that describes this policy should be available for patients to review.

[1]Defined herein as physicians, dentists, and podiatrists.

Proper provider credentials are also emphasized by the ASA in the accompanying *Statement on Qualifications of Anesthesia Providers in the Office-Based Setting* that was approved by the House of Delegates in the same year (3). It stresses that "specific anesthesia training for supervising operating practitioners and other licensed physicians" is especially important in an office-based environment where clinical resources may be limited and emergency facilities may not be readily available. The guidelines for qualifications of anesthesia providers are straightforward, the focus being patient safety and high quality of care. A person extensively trained in the delivery of anesthesia should be involved. If that person is not a physician, then a physician should directly supervise the patient's anesthesia care. Because there has been much discussion about who can and who cannot perform anesthesia in the office-based setting, this statement, shown in Box 5.3, emphasizes proper provider training and appropriate supervision.

Box 5.3

Various ASA policy documents, including the "Guidelines for Ambulatory Anesthesia and Surgery," contemplate that all anesthetics will be delivered by or under the medical direction of an anesthesiologist. ASA recognizes, however, that Medicare regulations and the laws or regulations of virtually all states contemplate that where anesthesiologist participation is not practicable, non-physician anesthesia providers must at minimum be supervised by the operating practitioner or other licensed physician.

ASA believes that anesthesiologist participation in all office-based surgery is optimally desirable as an important anesthesia patient safety standard, and it will always support such a standard. It does not oppose regulatory requirements that, where necessary, speak merely in terms of "physician" supervision. Those requirements should, however, require that the supervising physician be specifically trained in sedation, anesthesia, and rescue techniques appropriate to the type of sedation or anesthesia being provided as well as being trained in the office-based surgery performed.

ASA believes that specific anesthesia training for supervising physicians, while important in all anesthetizing locations, is especially critical in connection with office-based surgery where normal institutional back up or emergency facilities and capacities are often not available.

Since OBA is considered a subspecialty within ambulatory anesthesia, the *Guidelines for Ambulatory Anesthesia and Surgery*, first approved by the ASA House of Delegates in 1973 and reaffirmed in 2003, should also be adhered to. It addresses the need for adequate professional (physicians, nurses) as well as administrative, housekeeping, and maintenance staffing. It also calls for *"established policies and procedures"* to deal with medical emergencies and patient transfers (2).

FACILITY AND SAFETY

The second part of the Guidelines for Office-Based Anesthesia refers to facility management (see Box 5.4). Many office-based facilities have limited regulation other than that pertaining to fire and equipment safety, building and occupancy codes, occupational safety, and waste (such as anesthetic gas) disposal. In addition, there are state and federal laws governing distribution and storage of controlled substances that should be taken into consideration.

Box 5.4

The Guidelines for Office-Based Anesthesia Based on Facility Management
- Facilities should comply with all applicable federal, state, and local laws, codes, and regulations pertaining to:
  - Fire prevention
  - Building construction and occupancy
  - Accommodations for the disabled
  - Occupational safety and health
  - Disposal of medical waste and hazardous waste
- Policies and procedures should comply with laws and regulations pertaining to controlled drug supply, storage, and administration.

The *Guidelines for Nonoperating Room Anesthetizing Locations* were first approved by the ASA House of Delegates in 1994, and last amended in 2003 (4). They were passed at a time when the anesthesiology profession recognized the rapid growth of OBA and the need for recommendations to improve patient safety and improve quality. They address issues that are often taken for granted at large acute care hospitals: the need for reliable oxygen and suction sources, a gas scavenging system, adequate electric power and lightning, sufficient office space for equipment and personnel, and the availability of an emergency cart. It is suggested that in each location there should be the following:

- A reliable source of oxygen adequate for the length of the procedure
- A backup supply
- An adequate and reliable source of suction—a suction apparatus that meets operating room standards

Before administering any anesthetic, the anesthesiologist should consider the capabilities, limitations, and accessibility of both the primary and backup oxygen sources. Oxygen piped from a central source, meeting applicable codes, is strongly encouraged. The backup system should include the equivalent of at least a full E cylinder.

- In any location in which inhalation anesthetics are administered, there should be an adequate and reliable system for scavenging waste anesthetic gases.

The Guidelines for Nonoperating Room Anesthetizing Locations continue with further recommendations addressing the need for adequate airway and drug supplies, and appropriate monitoring equipment (see Box 5.5) (4).

Box 5.5

In each location, there should be the following:

- Self-inflating hand resuscitator bag capable of administering at least 90% oxygen as a means to deliver positive pressure ventilation.
- Adequate anesthesia drugs, supplies, and equipment for the intended anesthesia care; and adequate monitoring equipment to allow adherence to the "Standards for Basic Anesthetic Monitoring."
- Anesthesia machine equivalent in function to that employed in operating rooms and maintained to current operating room standards for inhalation anesthesia to be administered.
- Sufficient electrical outlets to satisfy anesthesia machine and monitoring equipment requirements, including clearly labeled outlets connected to an emergency power supply; either isolated electric power or electric circuits with ground fault circuit interrupters in any anesthetizing location determined by the health care facility to be a "wet location" (e.g., for cystoscopy or arthroscopy or a birthing room in labor and delivery).
- Provision for adequate illumination of the patient, anesthesia machine (when present) and monitoring equipment; in addition, a form of battery-powered illumination other than a laryngoscope should be immediately available.
- Expeditious access to the patient, anesthesia machine (when present) and monitoring equipment.
- An emergency cart with a defibrillator, emergency drugs, and other equipment adequate to provide cardiopulmonary resuscitation.
- Adequate staff trained to support the anesthesiologist and reliable means of two-way communication to request assistance.

PATIENT AND PROCEDURE SELECTION

There are two major issues that the anesthesiologist needs to address before initiating an anesthetic in the office. The first question is whether the patient would be an *appropriate* candidate for the proposed procedure. The second question is whether the type of the proposed surgical procedure would be *appropriate* for an office-based setting (5–7).

The *ASA Guidelines for Office-Based Anesthesia* state that, "*Patients who by reason of pre-existing medical or other conditions may be at undue risk for complications should be referred to an appropriate facility for performance of the procedure and the administration of anesthesia* (1)." However, it does not offer any specific criteria for patient selection. The *ASA Basic Standards for Preanesthesia Care* should, of course, apply to all patients being considered for OBA. This includes a preoperative interview, review of medical and anesthetic history and relevant laboratory results and studies, a focused physician examination, and the obtaining of an informed consent. The provider in the office is responsible for the following:

- *Reviewing the available medical record*
- *Interviewing and performing a focused examination of the patient to discuss the medical history, including previous anesthetic experiences and medical therapy and to assess those aspects of the patient's physical condition that might affect decisions regarding perioperative risk and management*
- *Ordering and reviewing pertinent available tests and consultations as necessary for the delivery of anesthesia care*
- *Ordering appropriate preoperative medications*
- *Ensuring that consent has been obtained for the anesthesia care*
- *Documenting in the chart that the above has been performed*

Many offices establish their own specific guidelines for patient and procedure selection. In the recently published work, *Office-Based Anesthesia: Considerations for Anesthesiologists in Setting Up and Maintaining a Safe Office Anesthesia Environment* (6), the authors suggested taking specific patient factors into consideration when deciding whether he or she may be an appropriate candidate:

1. Abnormalities of major organ systems, and stability and optimization of any medical illness
2. Difficult airway
3. Previous adverse experience with anesthesia and surgery
4. Current medications and drug allergies
5. Time and nature of the last oral intake
6. History of alcohol or substance use or abuse
7. Presence of an adult who assumes responsibility specifically for caring for and accompanying the patient from the office

Not all surgical procedures may be appropriate for an office-based setting. The *Guidelines for OBA* clearly state that the anesthesiologist needs to make sure that the "*procedure to be undertaken is within the scope of practice of the health care practitioners*" as well as "*capabilities of the facility.*" Furthermore, "*the procedure should be of a duration and degree of complexity that will permit the patient to recover and be discharge from the facility.*" Only a few states have specific regulations governing the types of procedures appropriate for an office. Many facilities must establish their own criteria for patient and procedure selection. It is important to realize that some surgical procedures may require a prolonged postanesthesia recovery, may delay discharge, or may be too complex to be performed in the office (examples include intra-abdominal, intrathoracic and intracranial procedures).

PERIOPERATIVE CARE

Several ASA documents address preoperative, intraoperative and postoperative care, and the same standards should apply to any OBA practice. For a thorough understanding of these guidelines, it is important to review the ASA documents listed in Box 5.6.

Box 5.6

Basic Standards for Pre-Anesthesia Care
Standards for Basic Anesthetic Monitoring
Guidelines for Ambulatory Anesthesia and Surgery
Statement on the Anesthesia Care Team
Standards for Post-Anesthesia Care

In 1999, the ASA House of Delegates approved the *Continuum of Depth of Sedation—Definition of General Anesthesia and Levels of Sedation / Analgesia* (8). This document defined four levels of sedation (minimal sedation/anxiolysis, moderate sedation/analgesia, deep sedation/analgesia, and general anesthesia) and these definitions were also adopted by the Joint Commission on Accreditation of Healthcare Organizations (JCAHO) as standards (see Table 5.1).

Minimal sedation (anxiolysis) is a drug-induced state during which patients respond normally to verbal commands. Although cognitive function and coordination may be impaired, ventilatory and cardiovascular functions are unaffected.

Moderate sedation / analgesia ("conscious sedation") is a drug-induced depression of consciousness during which patients respond purposefully[2] to verbal commands, either alone or accompanied by light tactile stimulation. No interventions are required to maintain a patent airway, and spontaneous ventilation is adequate. Cardiovascular function is usually maintained.

Deep sedation / analgesia is a drug-induced depression of consciousness during which patients cannot be easily aroused but respond purposefully (reflex withdrawal from a painful stimulus is NOT considered a purposeful response) following repeated or painful stimulation. The ability to independently maintain ventilatory function may be impaired. Patients may require assistance in maintaining a patent airway, and spontaneous ventilation may be inadequate. Cardiovascular function is usually maintained.

General anesthesia is a drug-induced loss of consciousness during which patients are not arousable, even by painful stimulation. The ability to independently maintain ventilatory function is often impaired. Patients often require assistance in maintaining a patent airway, and positive pressure ventilation may be required because of depressed spontaneous ventilation or drug-induced depression of neuromuscular function. Cardiovascular function may be impaired.

The statement also states that, *"Because sedation is a continuum, it is not always possible to predict how an individual patient will respond. Hence, practitioners intending to produce a given level of sedation should be able to rescue[3] patients whose level of sedation becomes deeper than initially intended. Individuals administering Moderate Sedation / Analgesia ("Conscious Sedation") should be able to rescue patients who enter a state of Deep Sedation / Analgesia, while those administering Deep Sedation / Analgesia should be able to rescue patients who enter a state of General Anesthesia."*

The statement also refers to monitored anesthesia care (MAC) as follows (9):

Monitored Anesthesia Care does not describe the continuum of depth of sedation, rather it describes "a specific anesthesia service in which an anesthesiologist has been requested to participate in the care of a patient undergoing a diagnostic or therapeutic procedure.

[2]Reflex withdrawal from a painful stimulus is not considered a purposeful stimulus.

[3]Rescue of a patient from a deeper level of sedation than intended is an intervention by a practitioner proficient in airway management and advanced life support. The qualified practitioner corrects adverse physiologic consequences of the deeper-than-intended level of sedation (such as hypoventilation, hypoxia, and hypotension) and returns the patient to the originally intended level of sedation.

Table 5.1. Continuum of depth of sedation

	Minimal Sedation (Anxiolysis)	Moderate Sedation/ Analgesia ("Conscious Sedation)	Deep Sedation/ Analgesia	General Anesthesia
Responsiveness	Normal response to verbal stimulation	Purposeful response to verbal or tactile stimulation	Purposeful response following repeated or painful stimulation	Unarousable even with painful stimulation
Airway	Unaffected	No intervention required	Intervention may be required	Intervention often required
Spontaneous Ventilation	Unaffected	Adequate	May be inadequate	Frequently inadequate
Cardiovascular Function	Unaffected	Usually maintained	Usually maintained	May be impaired

In addition, another document passed by the ASA House of Delegates in 2004 attempts to distinguish MAC from moderate sedation/analgesia (i.e., conscious sedation). Specifically, *Distinguishing Monitored Anesthesia Care From Moderate Sedation/Analgesia* states that MAC is a "physician service" that is different from moderate sedation "due to the expectations and qualifications of the provider who must be able to utilize all anesthesia resources to support life and to provide patient comfort and safety during a diagnostic or therapeutic procedure (5)."

JCAHO also incorporated in its standards the need to be able to rescue patients from a deeper level of sedation, and introduced a requirement for an additional qualified individual to monitor the patient. This also appears as a recommendation in ASA's *"Practice Guidelines for Sedation and Analgesia by Non-Anesthesiologists."* Specifically, it addressed the need to have a health care provider other than the one performing the procedure to monitor the patient (10):

A designated individual, other than the practitioner performing the procedure, should be present to monitor the patient throughout procedures performed with sedation/analgesia. During deep sedation, this individual should have no other responsibilities. However, during moderate sedation, this individual may assist with minor, interruptible tasks once the patient's level of sedation/analgesia and vital signs have stabilized, provided that adequate monitoring for the patient's level of sedation is maintained.

Postanesthesia care is an integral part of the overall perioperative care of a patient undergoing an office-based procedure. The *Guidelines for Office-Based Anesthesia* clearly state that the anesthesiologist should be immediately available until the patient has been discharged form anesthesia care, and that discharge of the patient is a physician responsibility. It calls for proper documentation of postoperative events, and also calls for health care staff with training in advanced resuscitative techniques (advanced cardiac life support [ACLS], pediatric advanced life support [PALS]) to be "immediately available" until all patients are discharged home. The recovery criteria, types and frequency of postoperative monitoring, and the availability of trained personnel all need to be addressed. A set of useful guidelines, *Standards for Post-Anesthesia Care,* was last amended by the ASA House of Delegates in 2004. A brief summary of five basic standards are outlined in Box 5.7 (11).

Box 5.7

Standard I
All patients who have received general anesthesia, regional anesthesia, or monitored anesthesia care shall receive appropriate postanesthesia management.

Standard II
A patient transported to the postanesthesia care unit (PACU) shall be accompanied by a member of the anesthesia care team who is knowledgeable about the patient's condition. The patient shall be continually evaluated and treated during transport with monitoring and support appropriate to the patient's condition.

Standard III
Upon arrival in the PACU, the patient shall be re-evaluated and a verbal report provided to the responsible PACU nurse by the member of the anesthesia care team who accompanies the patient.

Standard IV
The patient's condition shall be evaluated continually in the PACU.

Standard V
A physician is responsible for the discharge of the patient from the PACU.

MONITORING

The *Guidelines for Office-Based Anesthesia* specifically address the need for proper perioperative monitoring of all patients receiving anesthesia. The document also refers to the ASA *Standards for Basic Anesthetic Monitoring*, which were first approved in 1986 and last amended by the ASA House of Delegates in 2005. Monitoring standards in the office-based setting should not differ from the standards used in an acute care hospital facility (12). The monitoring principles outlined in this document apply to all patients undergoing anesthesia in all kinds of facilities, including the office. Specifically, it addresses the monitoring of *oxygenation, ventilation, circulation*, and *body temperature*. Although these guidelines are applicable to hospital and office-based locations, compliance with these basic patient monitoring techniques becomes especially important in the office-based setting where equipment, supplies, and personnel are often limited. Some exceptions do apply, and some monitoring requirements may be waived by the anesthesiologist under special circumstances (marked by*). It is critical for every anesthesia provider to review these monitoring standards (see Box 5.8).

Box 5.8

Standard I
Qualified anesthesia personnel shall be present in the room throughout the conduct of all general anesthetics, regional anesthetics, and MAC. Because of the rapid changes in patient status during anesthesia, qualified anesthesia personnel shall be continuously present to monitor the patient and provide anesthesia care. In the event there is a direct known hazard, e.g., radiation, to the anesthesia personnel, which might require intermittent remote observation of the patient, some provision for monitoring the patient must be made. In the event that an emergency requires the temporary absence of the person primarily responsible for the anesthetic, the best judgment of the anesthesiologist will be exercised in comparing the emergency with the anesthetized patient's condition and in the selection of the person left responsible for the anesthetic during the temporary absence.

Standard II
During all anesthetics, the patient's oxygenation, ventilation, circulation, and temperature shall be continually evaluated.

Oxygenation
1. Inspired gas: During every administration of general anesthesia using an anesthesia machine, the concentration of oxygen in the patient breathing system shall be measured by an oxygen analyzer with a low oxygen concentration limit alarm in use.*
2. Blood oxygenation: During all anesthetics, a quantitative method of assessing oxygenation such as pulse oximetry shall be employed.* When the pulse oximeter is utilized, the variable pitch pulse tone and the low threshold alarm shall be audible to the anesthesiologist or the anesthesia care team personnel.* Adequate illumination and exposure of the patient are necessary to assess color.*

Ventilation
1. Every patient receiving general anesthesia shall have the adequacy of ventilation continually evaluated. Qualitative clinical signs such as chest excursion, observation of the reservoir breathing bag, and auscultation of breath sounds are useful. Continual monitoring for the presence of expired carbon dioxide shall be performed unless invalidated by the nature of the patient, procedure, or equipment. Quantitative monitoring of the volume of expired gas is strongly encouraged.*

Box 5.8 *Continued*

2. When an endotracheal tube or laryngeal mask is inserted, its correct positioning must be verified by clinical assessment and by identification of carbon dioxide in the expired gas. Continual end-tidal carbon dioxide analysis, in use from the time of endotracheal tube/laryngeal mask placement, until extubation/removal or initiating transfer to a postoperative care location, shall be performed using a quantitative method such as capnography, capnometry, or mass spectroscopy.* When capnography or capnometry is utilized, the end tidal CO_2 alarm shall be audible to the anesthesiologist or the anesthesia care team personnel.*

3. When ventilation is controlled by a mechanical ventilator, there shall be in continuous use a device that is capable of detecting disconnection of components of the breathing system. The device must give an audible signal when its alarm threshold is exceeded.

4. During regional anesthesia and MAC, the adequacy of ventilation shall be evaluated by continual observation of qualitative clinical signs and/or monitoring for the presence of exhaled carbon dioxide.

Circulation

1. Every patient receiving anesthesia shall have the electrocardiogram continuously displayed from the beginning of anesthesia until preparing to leave the anesthetizing location.*

2. Every patient receiving anesthesia shall have arterial blood pressure and heart rate determined and evaluated at least every 5 minutes.*

3. Every patient receiving general anesthesia shall have, in addition to the above, circulatory function continually evaluated by at least one of the following: palpation of a pulse, auscultation of heart sounds, monitoring of a tracing of intra-arterial pressure, ultrasound peripheral pulse monitoring, or pulse plethysmography or oximetry.

Body Temperature

Every patient receiving anesthesia shall have temperature monitored when clinically significant changes in body temperature are intended, anticipated, or suspected.

EQUIPMENT

As outlined in the ASA *Guidelines for Office-Based Anesthesia*, the following equipment-related issues need to be taken into consideration:

- All facilities should have a reliable source of oxygen, suction, resuscitation equipment, and emergency drugs. Specific reference is made to the ASA *Guidelines for Nonoperating Room Anesthetizing Locations* (*see* "Facility and Safety" for a review) (4).
- There should be sufficient space to accommodate all necessary equipment and personnel and to allow for expeditious access to the patient, anesthesia machine (when present), and all monitoring equipment.
- All equipment should be maintained, tested, and inspected according to the manufacturer's specifications.
- Backup power sufficient to ensure patient protection in the event of an emergency should be available.
- In any location in which anesthesia is administered, there should be appropriate anesthesia apparatus and equipment which allow monitoring consistent with ASA *Standards for Basic Anesthetic Monitoring* (*see* "Monitoring" for a review) and documentation of regular preventive maintenance as recommended by the manufacturer (12).

- In an office where anesthesia services are to be provided to infants and children, the required equipment, medication, and resuscitative capabilities should be appropriately sized for a pediatric population.

Another document that addresses the age of anesthesia equipment is the *ASA Guidelines for Determining Anesthesia Machine Obsolescence* developed by the ASA Committee on Equipment and Facilities (13). It is important to note that the age of the anesthesia machine alone may not automatically make it obsolete, and that the machine *"should not be expected to meet all of the performance and safety requirements after the machine was manufactured."* The current guidelines examine the gas and vapor delivery portions of the machine as criteria for defining machine obsolescence. For the *"absolute"* criteria, the document addresses the lack of essential safety features, such as O_2/N_2O proportioning system, pin index safety system, and oxygen supply pressure failure alarm. In addition, the presence of *"unacceptable features"* such as measure flow vaporizers and the inability to adequately maintain the machine are reasons for judging the machine obsolete.

EMERGENCIES AND TRANSFERS

The anesthesiologist and other health care providers must be properly trained and equipped to deal with all types of emergencies that may occasionally arise in office-based settings. Each facility must develop and regularly review emergency protocols, including mechanisms for a safe patient transfer to an acute care facility.

The *ASA Guidelines for Office-Based Anesthesia* emphasize the need for the following:

- Written protocols are necessary for cardiopulmonary emergencies and other internal and external disasters such as fire or flood.
- If the facility uses malignant hyperthermia-triggering agents, it must have medications and equipment available to treat the patient.
- The office facility must possess basic emergency medications and equipment necessary for cardiopulmonary resuscitation and for the initiation of ASA Difficult Airway Algorithm.
- The emphasis is on the same standard of care one would expect in an acute care facility or an outpatient surgicenter.
- It is also important to make sure that the health care provider must be trained in advanced life support and be immediately available until all patients are discharged home.

REFERENCES

1. American Society of Anesthesiologists. *Guidelines for office-based anesthesia.* (Approved by ASA House of Delegates; on October 13, 1999, and reaffirmed on October 27, 2004). Available at: www.asahq.org/publicationsAndServices/standards/12.pdf. 2004.
2. American Society of Anesthesiologists. *Guidelines for ambulatory anesthesia and surgery.* (Approved by ASA House of Delegates; on October 11, 1973, reaffirmed on October 15, 2003). Available at: www.asahq.org/publicationsAndServices/standards/04.pdf. 2003.
3. American Society of Anesthesiologists. *Statement on qualifications of anesthesia providers in the office-based setting.* (Approved by ASA House of Delegates; on October 13, 1999, last affirmed 2004). Available at: www.asahq.org/publicationsAndServices/standards/29.pdf. 2004.
4. American Society of Anesthesiologists. *Guidelines for nonoperating room anesthetizing locations.* (Approved by ASA House of Delegates; on October 19, 1994, amended on October 15, 2003). Available at: www.asahq.org/publicationsAndServices/standards/14.pdf. 2003.

5. American Society of Anesthesiologists. *Position on monitored anesthesia care.* (Approved by ASA House of Delegates; on October 21, 1986, amended on October 25, 2005). Available at: www.asahq.org/publicationsAndServices/standards/23.pdf. 2005.
6. ASA Committee on Ambulatory Surgical Care and ASA Task Force on Office-Based Anesthesia. *Office-based anesthesia: Considerations for anesthesiologists in setting up and maintaining a safe office anesthesia environment.* ASA Committee on Ambulatory Surgical Care and ASA Task Force on Office-Based Anesthesia; Available at: http://www.asahq.org/publicationsAndServices/office.pdf. 2002.
7. American Society of Anesthesiologists. *Statement on the anesthesia care team.* (Approved by ASA House of Delegates; on October 26, 1982, amended on October 17, 2001). Available at: www.asahq.org/publicationsAndServices/standards/16.pdf. 2001.
8. American Society of Anesthesiologists. *Continuum of depth of sedation definitions of general anesthesia and levels of sedation / analgesia.* (Approved by ASA House of Delegates; on October 13, 1999, amended October 27, 2004). Available at: www.asahq.org/publicationsAndServices/standards/20.pdf. 2004.
9. American Society of Anesthesiologists. *Distinguishing monitored anesthesia care ("MAC") from moderate sedation / analgesia-conscious sedation.* (Approved by the ASA House of Delegates; on October 27, 2004). Available at: www.asahq.org/publicationsAndServices/standards/35.pdf. 2004.
10. ASA Task Force on Sedation and Analgesia by Non-Anesthesiologists. Practice guidelines for sedation and analgesia by non-anesthesiologists (An updated report by the ASA Task Force on Sedation and Analgesia by Non-Anesthesiologists. *Anesthesiology.* 2002;96:1004–1017.
11. American Society of Anesthesiologists. *Standards for post-anesthesia care.* (Approved by ASA House of Delegates; on October 12, 1988, amended October 27, 2004). Available at: www.asahq.org/publicationsAndServices/standards/36.pdf. 2004.
12. American Society of Anesthesiologists. *Standards for basic anesthetic monitoring* (Approved by ASA House of Delegates; on October 21, 1986, amended October 25, 2005). Available at: www.asahq.org/publicationsAndServices/standards/02.pdf. 2005.
13. American Society of Anesthesiologists. *Guidelines for determining anesthesia machine obsolescence.* Available at: www.asahq.org/publicationsAndServices/machineobsolescense.pdf. 2006.

The Preoperative Evaluation

Richard D. Urman, Jonathan Kaper, and Fred E. Shapiro

A pleasant and comfortable outcome for the patient will begin with planning in advance of the surgery. Such planning includes reviewing the patient's medical history, scheduling the preoperative interview and physical examination, assessing for possible drug interactions with anesthetic, deciding on the most appropriate type of anesthesia, and then developing a complete care plan.

It is widely recognized that a thorough preoperative evaluation is a critical aspect of patient care. The anesthesiologist, however, is often faced with several issues that are unique to the office. More often than not, the anesthesiologist will meet and evaluate the patient on the day of the scheduled procedure. Therefore, although the patient would have been seen by the surgeon who would perform the initial patient evaluation, a focused preanesthetic evaluation would not have occurred. Unfortunately, the office usually does not have the traditional preoperative testing center now common in most hospitals. As the anesthesiologist evaluates the patient before providing anesthesia services, it is important to ask the following two questions:

> *Is the proposed procedure appropriate to be performed in the office?*
> *Is the patient a good candidate for the procedure to be performed in the office?*

There are procedures that may be inappropriate for an office-based setting. Many states and professional organizations have established rules and guidelines defining the complexity of surgical procedures and their appropriateness for an office-based setting. Some procedures may require nothing more than local anesthesia or conscious sedation, whereas others may require general anesthesia. When the anesthesiologist is evaluating the patient, it is important to consider how the proposed surgical procedure will impact the length of recovery and the complexity of postoperative care by the recovery room staff. Procedures that may entail large blood loss or large fluid shifts may not be appropriate for the office, as are procedures involving intracranial, intra-abdominal or intrathoracic cavities. The anesthesiologist must ascertain that the proposed procedure is within the scope of practice of the office facility and all health care providers involved (1).

PREOPERATIVE PATIENT EVALUATION

In addition to evaluating the appropriateness of the surgical procedure, the anesthesiologist must perform a thorough evaluation of the patient. In the office, this often takes place on the day of surgery, although ideally such an evaluation should take place days ahead to allow for necessary testing and medical record evaluation. Many offices begin by giving out a patient information packet, which includes an anesthesia information sheet. This handout provides answers to most frequently asked questions and addresses most common patient concerns (see Figure 6.1).

PREOPERATIVE INTERVIEW

To establish a good rapport with the patient and achieve a comfortable operating room experience, the nurse and/or anesthesiologist will interview

Name:	(Last, First)
Date of Birth:	(Month, Date, Year)
Marital Status:	(Married, Single, Divorced)
Occupation:	
Illnesses:	List any illnesses that requires medical attention
Hospitalizations:	Include dates, place, and reason
Surgical History:	Include operations and dates
Anesthesia:	Any problems with anesthesia in the past?
Allergies:	List drugs or any other substances any type of reaction
Injuries:	List any injuries you have had
Medications:	Include dosage and purpose
Habits:	*Tobacco* (amount and duration)
	Alcohol (type and amount used)
	Recreational drug use (list type/frequency)
Family History:	List medical problems that run in your family, including bleeding tendencies, inherited diseases, problems with anesthesia)
Review of Systems:	*General:*
	State of Health: Excellent, Good, Fair, Poor
	Recent Weight Change: Gain, Loss. How much?
	Eyes, ears, nose, throat, sinuses:
	Respiratory: Shortness of breath, mucous production, coughing up blood, wheezing, asthma
	Heart: Chest pain, high blood pressure, ankle swelling, awake at night, shortness of breath
	Gastrointestinal: Abdominal pain, change in bowel, habits, black stool, nausea, vomiting, history of jaundice, hepatitis, heartburn (reflux)
	Genitourinary: Kidney or bladder problems, trouble urinating, age of onset of periods, last menstrual period
	Musculoskeletal: Bone or joint trouble, weakeness, muscle disease history
	Nervous System: Seizures, fainting, headaches, dizziness, double vision, depression
	Endocrine: Diabetes, thyroid disease, adrenal problems
	Hematopoietic System: Anemia, bruise easily, bleeding tendencies

Figure 6.1.   Patient questionnaire.

the patient by either a telephone call or at an office visit. This is a way to get introduced to the patient and in an unhurried interview to discuss the anticipated plan of care. This way, any questions regarding the patient's medical history can be addressed, and any concerns of the patient can be discussed. These interviews are designed to ensure the goals of a safe and pleasant surgical and anesthetic experience are met, and to assure patients that their special concerns will be addressed. It is important for the anesthesia provider to alleviate the psychological stress of surgery by answering all of the patient's questions and being available if further patient concerns arise before surgery.

STANDARDS FOR ANESTHESIA CARE

In conjunction with various state and society regulations, many offices establish their own preoperative patient selection and evaluation guidelines.

Patient selection and evaluation criteria must also meet the standards set forth by the American Society of Anesthesiologists (ASA). The evaluation of patients for anesthesia in the office-based setting is further complicated by the fact that the resources taken for granted in the hospital-based operating room may not be immediately available. Careful classification of these patients must be performed to insure that they are indeed appropriate candidates for office-based anesthesia. The ASA has established *Basic Standards For Preanesthesia Care* (2), which were first approved by the ASA House of Delegates in 1987, and last amended in 2005. Specifically, these guidelines state that the anesthesiologist must review medical records, perform an appropriate physical examination, document relevant medical history, request additional testing and premedications, and obtain an informed consent. These recommendations describe the responsibilities of the anesthesiologist (see Box 6.1).

Box 6.1

The anesthesiologist, before the delivery of anesthesia care, is responsible for the following:

1. Reviewing the available medical record
2. Interviewing and performing a focused examination of the patient to:
   a. discuss the medical history, including previous anesthetic experiences and medical therapy
   b. assess those aspects of the patient's physical condition that might affect decisions regarding perioperative risk and management
3. Ordering and reviewing pertinent available tests and consultations as necessary for the delivery of anesthesia
4. Ordering appropriate preoperative medications
5. Ensuring that consent has been obtained for the anesthesia care
6. Documenting in the chart that the above has been performed

---

These standards apply to all patients who receive anesthesia or monitored anesthesia care, and the anesthesiologist should be responsible for "determining the medical status of the patient" and "developing a plan of anesthesia care." Under unusual circumstances (e.g., extreme emergencies), these standards may be modified. When this is the case, the circumstances shall be documented in the patient's record. The ASA physical status classification is also used to standardize the way patients are categorized (ASA I-VI) based on pre-existing medical condition (see Box 6.2). This classification system has been used as a common denominator for all communication, guidelines, discussion, and research purposes. In evaluating patients for surgery, the anesthesiologist and the office staff should pay a particularly close attention to the ASA Class III and IV patients who may require optimization of their medical conditions before surgery or may not be appropriate candidates for office surgery.

Box 6.2

ASA Physical Status Classification Guidelines
P1   Normal healthy patient
P2   Patient with mild systemic disease
P3   Patient with severe systemic disease
P4   Patient with severe systemic disease that is a constant threat to life
P5   Moribund patient who is not expected to survive without the operation
P6   Declared brain-dead patient whose organs are being removed for donor purposes

---

If the patient has had anesthesia in the past, it is important to note previous problems with anesthesia as well as good experiences in order to better tailor the anesthetic plan for each individual patient. In addition, a family history of problems with anesthesia must also be obtained.

The history and physical examination are the best measures of screening for disease and should be completed well in advance of the surgery. A patient-completed questionnaire will assist the surgeon and anesthesiologist in determining the need for further workup. Special attention should be paid to predictors of perioperative cardiac morbidity such as history of previous myocardial infarction, congestive heart failure, angina, hypertension, diabetes, cardiac arrhythmias, peripheral vascular disease, valvular heart disease, cigarette smoking, and obesity. The anesthesiologist should follow the current American College of Cardiology/American Heart Association guidelines for perioperative cardiovascular testing for noncardiac surgery (3).

In all patients, pertinent laboratory values and test results (hematology and chemistry laboratories, electrocardiogram, chest x-ray, cardiac/pulmonary reports) must be evaluated and reviewed by the anesthesiologist before the procedure. In addition, it may be necessary to obtain further tests and consultations that will be necessary to conduct the anesthesia. Before undergoing anesthesia, the patient may need medical clearance or may need comorbid conditions optimized before surgery. The history and physical examination should be current and re-evaluated by the surgeon on the day of surgery to ascertain that no significant changes in medical condition have occurred.

Despite these interventions, some patients may still not be good candidates for an elective cosmetic procedure that is to be performed in an office-based setting. It is important to assess these situations in advance to avoid canceling a procedure based on a lack of preoperative preparation. Because these preexisting conditions have the potential for perioperative problems, patients with unstable conditions should be referred to a hospital where their specific medical conditions can be managed more acutely. As with any health care matter, it is important for the patient to be involved in the planning and the delivery of their care.

While performing a preoperative evaluation, the anesthesiologist should take the following factors into consideration when deciding whether the patient may be an appropriate candidate for surgery (4):

Abnormalities of major organ systems
Stability and optimization of any medical illness
Difficult airway
Previous adverse experience with anesthesia and surgery
Current medications and drug allergies
Time and nature of the last oral intake
History of alcohol or substance use or abuse
Presence of an adult who assumes responsibility specifically for caring for and accompanying the patient from the office

Preoperative preparation should also include adherence to the NPO guidelines outlined in the *ASA Practice Guidelines for Preoperative Fasting* (see Table 6.1) (5). These should apply to all patients in all settings. Many experts suggest the following NPO guidelines for patients undergoing surgery. Such guidelines generally apply to all ages, and are particularly useful for healthy patients undergoing elective procedures.

PREOPERATIVE TESTING

Although much has been written about preoperative testing, there is no conclusive evidence about routine testing. The *ASA Task Force on Perioperative Testing* (6) concluded that preoperative tests should not be ordered routinely, but rather on a selective basis for "purposes of guiding or optimizing perioperative management." Therefore, indications for preoperative

Table 6.1. NPO guidelines for preoperative fasting

	Minimum Fasting Period (h)
Clear Liquids	2
Breast Milk	4
Infant Formula	6
Nonhuman Milk	6
Light Meal	6
Meat, fried/fatty foods	8

From: Warner MA, Caplan RA, Epstein BS, et al. The Task Force on Preoperative Fasting and the Use of Pharmacologic Agents to Reduce the Risk of Pulmonary Aspiration. Practice guidelines for preoperative fasting and the use of pharmacologic agents to reduce the risk of pulmonary aspiration: Application to healthy patients undergoing elective procedures: A Report by the American Society of Anesthesiologists Task Force on Preoperative Fasting. *Anesthesiology.* 1999;90(3):896–905.

testing should be documented in the patient's chart and based on the information available in the chart, physical examination, and interview, the type of procedure should be planned. The task force developed a chart based on surveys of anesthesia consultants and ASA members. For selected patients, the patient characteristics found in Table 6.2 may warrant additional preoperative testing.

PREPARING FOR DRUG AND DIETARY SUPPLEMENT INTERACTIONS WITH ANESTHESIA

Anesthetic agents may interact with dietary supplements and herbal remedies. It is important to know how prescription drugs, nonprescription drugs, herbal supplements, and dietary supplements each interact with anesthesia. Drug interactions with anesthetic agents are an important concern to anesthesiologists because these interactions may make it difficult to maintain the patient's stable medical condition and also affect the amount of anesthesia required during the perioperative period.

Some medications may be taken but others should either be discontinued before surgery or additional caution must be exercised. Table 6.3 may be used as an aid to determine the appropriate preoperative medications and how these medications will interact with anesthetic agents.

HERBAL MEDICATIONS

The effects of herbal medications and dietary supplements on anesthesia are somewhat controversial. The U.S. Food and Drug Administration (FDA) has not specifically delineated these substances as "drugs," unless the product label on these substances implicitly claims to treat, diagnose, prevent, or cure a disease. In that case, the substance must then meet the safety and effectiveness standards under the Food, Drug, and Cosmetic Act. In April 1998, the FDA issued "regulations on statements made for dietary supplements concerning the effects of the product on the structure and function of the body." To circumvent FDA drug regulation, the manufacturers of the various products have placed the terms "this is not intended to diagnose, treat, prevent, or cure a disease." Based on this current controversy and the concern for these herbal and dietary supplements to interact with anesthetic medications and surgery, the ASA states that it

takes no formal position on the therapeutic properties of herbal medications and has no formal statement of policy or standard of care that is specific to phytopharmaceuticals (7).

Table 6.2. Patient characteristics for selected preoperative testing

Preoperative Test	Patient Characteristics	Consultants ($n = 72$)	ASA Members ($n = 234$)
Electrocardiogram	Advanced age	93%	94%
	Cardiocirculatory disease	97%	98%
	Respiratory disease	74%	74%
Other cardiac evaluation (e.g., stress test)	Cardiovascular compromise	88%	95%
Chest radiograph	Recent upper respiratory infection	45%	59%
	Smoking	42%	60%
	COPD	71%	76%
	Cardiac disease	62%	75%
Pulmonary function tests	Reactive airway disease	68%	71%
	COPD	80%	89%
	Scoliosis	53%	60%
Office spirometry (i.e., portable spirometer)	Reactive airway disease	83%	86%
	COPD	77%	90%
	Scoliosis	51%	52%
Hemoglobin/hematocrit	Advanced age	57%	68%
	Very young age	52%	56%
	Anemia	96%	99%
	Bleeding disorders	93%	94%
	Other hematological disorders	74%	84%
Coagulation studies	Bleeding disorders	99%	98%
	Renal dysfunction	40%	52%
	Liver dysfunction	97%	91%
	Anticoagulants	97%	96%
Serum chemistries (sodium, potassium, carbon dioxide, chloride, glucose)	Endocrine disorders	93%	95%
	Renal dysfunction	96%	98%
	Medications	87%	89%
Pregnancy test	Uncertain pregnancy history	84%	91%
	History suggestive of current pregnancy	94%	96%

ASA, American Society of Anesthesiologists; COPD, chronic obstructive pulmonary disease.
From: Pasternak LR, Arens JF, Caplan RA, et al. Task Force on Preanesthesia Evaluation. Practice advisory for preanesthesia evaluation: A report by the American Society of Anesthesiologists Task Force on Preanesthesia Evaluation. *Anesthesiology.* 2002;96(2):485–496.

Table 6.3. Preoperative medications and their interaction with anesthetic agents

Drug Class	Preoperative Preparation	Potential Intraoperative Problems
Antianginal	Sublingual tablets can be continued until induction with IV nitroglycerin or paste administered intraoperatively as needed	Potentiation of hypotensive effects of some anesthetic agents, particularly in hypovolemic patients
Antiarrhythmics	Continue to day of surgery	Some may potentiate neuromuscular blockers
Antibiotics	Discuss perioperative antibiotic management with surgeon	Aminoglycosides potentiate neuromuscular blockers
Antidiabetic	Measure preoperative blood sugar preoperatively; continue oral hypoglycemic until day of surgery; consider reducing insulin dose	Intraoperative fluctuations in blood sugar
Antihypertensives	Continue to day of surgery	Potentiation of hypotensive effects of some anesthetic agents, particularly in hypovolemic patients
Antiparkinsonian	Continue levodopa until the night before surgery	Phenothiazines may counteract antiparkinson effects of levodopa.
Antiseizure medications	Continue phenytoin and phenobarbital to day of surgery	Phenytoin may augment nondepolarizing neuromuscular blockade
β-Blockers	Continue to day of surgery	May potentiate cardiac depressant effects of some anesthetics
Cardiac glycosides	Continue to day of surgery; assess patient for signs digitalis toxicity or potassium depletion and correct if present	May potentiate nondepolarizing neuromuscular blockade
Corticosteroids	Generally continue steroids to day of surgery; may inhibit proper healing	Patient may require intraoperative and postoperative steroid supplementation depending on dose taken/duration of use
Psychotropes	Continue tricyclic antidepressants, lithium, phenothiazines, and antipsychotic to day of surgery	MAO inhibitors interact with narcotic analgesics, local anesthetic/epinephrine combinations and other vasopressors; lithium may prolong the effect of depolarizing muscle relaxants

MAO, monoamine oxidase.

The ASA also believes that it is important to make the public and the medical community

aware that these products could pose a serious health risk if they are taken prior to surgery. People often believe that a product that is labeled 'all natural' must therefore be safe. This is an inaccurate and dangerous assumption that can put patients at unnecessary risk (7).

The use of herbal medicines may be associated with physiologic changes that can result in perioperative complications. One recent study looked at the effect of common herbal medicines on perioperative events. The authors enrolled 601 patients, 80% of whom took self-prescribed herbal medicines such as licorice, ginkgo, ginger, ginseng, garlic, and other traditional Chinese herbs (8). Side effects included prolonged activated partial thromboplastin time and hypokalemia discovered preoperatively. They concluded that the use of traditional Chinese herbal medicines near the time of surgery should be discouraged because of the increased risk of adverse events in the preoperative period. It is also important to elicit information from the patient about the use of herbal medicines as it is the first step toward preventing and treating complications in the perioperative period. Many patients fail to reveal herbal medicine use during preoperative evaluations. Another potential problem is that herbal medicines are not regulated by the FDA and, consequently, do not have to meet the safety and efficacy requirements of regulated drugs. Adverse events stemming from herbal medication use are rarely reported because there is no standardized procedure for doing so. Although the ASA currently does not have a practice guideline concerning herbal medicine use and perioperative care, it distributed the following statement in its brochure, *Considerations for Anesthesiologists* (7):

> Use of herbs and other dietary supplements is not necessarily a contraindication to anesthesia. Pending more definitive studies and in the best interest of patient safety, the ASA is taking a leading role in educating the physician as well as the patient about the importance of a thorough history of a patient's medication use. Patients should tell their physicians—and physicians should ask—about all herbal, dietary, or other over-the-counter preparations as well as prescription medicine that they are taking.

There are thousands of herbal products and dietary supplements currently in the market. Listed in Table 6.4 are examples of some commonly used herbal and dietary products and their possible drug interactions (9).

CONCLUSION

A careful patient evaluation and preparation is key to a safe and mutually acceptable anesthetic plan. Preoperative evaluation is an integral part of patient care, and the standards and guidelines that apply to patients treated in acute care facilities should also apply to patients in an office-based setting. A preoperative patient interview, review of testing and medical record data, and a focused physical examination should be completed by the anesthesiologist before providing care. One must remember that part of the positive experience for the patient is an adequate preoperative evaluation, along with education about what to expect from the anesthesia and surgery. Hopefully, a patient who is well informed will be less anxious, may require less anesthesia, and may recover more rapidly. Intraoperative and postoperative care shall be discussed in a later chapter. It is important to realize that what makes the entire experience a positive one is the continuum of care from the preoperative assessment until the patient is healed—not simply during the period of time that he or she is in the operating room.

Table 6.4. Clinically important effects and perioperative concerns of eight herbal medicines and recommendations for discontinuation of use before surgery

Herb: Common Name(s)	Relevant Pharmacologic Effects	Perioperative Concerns	Preoperative Discontinuation
Echinacea: purple coneflower root	Activation of cell-mediated immunity	Allergic reactions: decreased effectiveness of immunosuppressants: potential for immunosuppression with long-term use	No data
Ephedra: ma huang	Increased heart rate and blood pressure through direct and indirect sympathomimetic effects	Risk of myocardial ischemia and stroke from tachycardia and hypertension, ventricular anhythmias with halothane: long-term use depletes endogenous catecholamines and may cause intraoperative hemodynamic instability; life-threatening interaction with monoamine oxidase inhibitors	At least 24 h before surgery
Garlic: ajo	Inhibition of platelet aggregation (may be irreversible); increased fibrinolysis; equivocal antihypertensive activity	Potential to increase risk of bleeding, especially when combined with other medications that inhibit platelet aggregation	At least 7 d before surgery
Ginkgo: duck foot tree, maidenhair tree, silver apricot	Inhibition of platelet-activating factor	Potential to increase risk of bleeding, especially when combined with other medications that inhibit platelet aggregation	At least 36 h before surgery

(continued)

Table 6.4. *(Continued)*

Herb: Common Name(s)	Relevant Pharmacologic Effects	Perioperative Concerns	Preoperative Discontinuation
Ginseng: American ginseng, Asian ginseng, Chinese ginseng, Korean ginseng	Lowers blood glucose; inhibition of platelet aggregation (may be irreversible); increased PT-PTT in animals; many other diverse effects	Hypoglycemia: potential to increase risk of bleeding; potential to decrease anticoagulation effect of warfarin	At least 7 d before surgery
Kava: awa, intoxicating pepper, kawa	Sedation, anxiolysis	Potential to increase sedative effect of anesthetics; potential for addiction, tolerance, and withdrawal after abstinence unstudied	At least 24 h before surgery
St John's wort; amber, goat weed, hardhay, Hypericum, Klamath weed	Inhibition of neurotransmitter reuptake, monoamine oxidase inhibition is unlikely	Induction of cytochrome P-450 enzymes, affecting cyclosporine, warfarin, steroids, protease inhibitors, and possibly benzodiazepines, calcium channel blockers, and many other drugs; decreased serum digoxin levels	At least 5 d before surgery
Valerian: all heal, garden heliotrope, vandal root	Sedation	Potential to increase sedative effect of anesthetics; benzodiazepine-like-acute withdrawal; potential to increase anesthetic requirements with long-term use	No data

PT, Prothrombin time; PTT, partial thromboplastin time.
From: Ang-Lee MK, Moss J, Yuan CS. Herbal medicines and perioperative care. *J Am Med Assoc.* 2001;286(2):208–216.

REFERENCES

1. American Society of Anesthesiologists. *Guidelines for office-based anesthesia.* Approved by ASA House of Delegates; on October 13, 1999, and last affirmed on October 27, 2004. Available at: www.asahq.org/publicationsAndServices/standards/12.pdf. 2004.
2. American Society of Anesthesiologists. *Basic standards for preanesthesia care.* Approved by the ASA House of Delegates; on October 14, 1987, and amended October 25, 2005. Available at: www.asahq.org/publicationsAndServices/standards/03.pdf. 2005.
3. Eagle KA, Berker PB, Calkins H, et al. ACC/AHA guideline update for perioperative cardiovascular evaluation for noncardiac surgery—executive summary. A report of the American College of Cardiology/American Heart Association Task Force on Practice Guideline. *Anest Analg.* 2002;94(5):1052–1064.
4. American Society of Anesthesiologists. *Office-based anesthesia: Considerations for anesthesiologists in setting up and maintaining a safe office anesthesia environment (ASA Committee on Ambulatory Surgical Care and ASA Task Force on Office-Based Anesthesia).* Available at: http://www.asahq.org/publicationsAndServices/office.pdf. 2002.
5. Warner MA, Caplan RA, Epstein BS, et al. The Task Force on Preoperative Fasting and the Use of Pharmacologic Agents to Reduce the Risk of Pulmonary Aspiration. Practice guidelines for preoperative fasting and the use of pharmacologic agents to reduce the risk of pulmonary aspiration: Application to healthy patients undergoing elective procedures: A Report by the American Society of Anesthesiologists Task Force on Preoperative Fasting. *Anesthesiology.* 1999;90(3):896–905.
6. Pasternak LR, Arens JF, Caplan RA, et al. Task Force on Preanesthesia Evaluation. Practice advisory for preanesthesia evaluation: A report by the American Society of Anesthesiologists Task Force on Preanesthesia Evaluation. *Anesthesiology.* 2002;96:485–496.
7. American Society of Anesthesiologists. *Considerations for anesthesiologists: What you should know about your patients' use of herbal medicines and other dietary supplements.* American Society of Anesthesiologists Brochure; Available at: www.asahq.org/patientEducation/herbPhysician.pdf. © 2003.
8. Lee A, Chiu PT, Aun CST, et al. Incidence and risk of adverse perioperative events among surgical patients taking traditional Chinese herbal medicines. *Anesthesiology.* 2006;105(3):454–461.
9. Ang-Lee MK, Moss J, Yuan CS. Herbal medicines and perioperative care. *J Am Med Assoc.* 2001;286(2):208–216.

Anesthesia Techniques: Which is the Safest Choice?

Richard D. Urman and Fred E. Shapiro

As anesthesia providers, we are often asked two simple questions:

1. *What type of anesthesia would you recommend?*
2. *Which is the safest choice?*

After reading this chapter, the reader will understand that these questions are not easy to answer.

The discussion concerning anesthetic safety in the office has been divided into two parts. The goal is to discuss a variety of anesthetic techniques that can be employed in an office setting, followed by a discussion of safety issues surrounding office-based anesthesia (OBA) practice. The chapter will conclude with a brief overview of the most recent literature addressing OBA safety.

THE CHOICE OF ANESTHESIA

It is important to realize that the same anesthetic techniques that are used in acute care hospitals and ambulatory surgical centers can be used in an office-based setting. The four broad categories are:

- Local anesthesia
- Monitored anesthesia care (MAC)
- Regional anesthesia
- General anesthesia

Techniques involving a combination of two or more of the anesthetic types have also been successfully used in the office. The anesthetic techniques are:

Local Anesthesia

This technique provides a loss of sensation to an area of the body. It is often used as the only anesthetic for a variety of procedures. Dermatologists, dentists, gastroenterologists, and surgeons have successfully used local anesthesia without the need for an anesthesiologist. Local anesthesia can also be used as an adjunct to monitored or general anesthesia, as well as for postoperative pain control.

Monitored Anesthesia Care

This technique involves the administration of medications that produce sedation and relieve pain. During the surgery, the patient's vital signs, which include the heart rate, blood pressure, respiratory rate, and oxygen level, are monitored in order to maintain stability and avoid sudden changes or complications. According to the American Society of Anesthesiologists (ASA), MAC may include varying levels of sedation, analgesia, and anxiolysis. Refer to the ASA guidelines regarding MAC anesthesia listed in the subsequent text.

Regional Anesthesia

Regional anesthesia techniques have been successfully used in office settings, and include spinal, epidural, and extremity nerve blocks. Spinal or epidural blocks are useful as sole anesthetics or can be employed in conjunction with MAC or general anesthesia. Various upper and lower extremity blocks can provide excellent intra- and postoperative analgesia.

General Anesthesia

This involves the loss of consciousness, lack of pain sensation, and purposeful response to stimuli. General anesthesia can be provided safely in the office by the anesthesiologist as long as proper equipment and monitoring are available (see Chapter 5).

Clearly, the choice of the anesthetic technique largely depends on the patient's medical condition, type of operation, as well as skills and training of the personneladministering anesthesia.

There is a fine line between sedation, deep sedation, and general anesthesia. Consumption of alcohol, recreational drug use, sensitivity to pain, and unusual reactions to medication (sometimes people have a decreased, increased, or opposite effect of what the drug is intended to do or perhaps an allergic reaction to a drug) may be crucial factors determining the most safe anesthetic technique for any particular patient.

An anesthetic plan ideally should be formulated before the patient's arrival to the office for surgery, after resolving any medical issues, and after having completed the necessary preoperative workup. These standards are the same regardless of the site where anesthesia is being administered.

The ASA *Guidelines for Office-Based Anesthesia* (1), which were last reaffirmed by the House of Delegates in 2004, outline the recommendations regarding clinical care and patient and procedure selection (see Box 7.1).

Box 7.1

Clinical Care Patient and Procedure Selection

- The anesthesiologist should be satisfied that the procedure to be undertaken is within the scope of practice of the health care practitioners and the capabilities of the facility.

- The procedure should be of a duration and degree of complexity that will permit the patient to recover and be discharged from the facility.

- Patients who by reason of pre-existing medical or other conditions may be at undue risk for complications should be referred to an appropriate facility for performance of the procedure and the administration of anesthesia.

Office-based surgery can offer medical care in a convenient, comfortable, and affordable environment. It is important to have the patient involved in the planning and delivery of care. Being informed and asking the right questions before undergoing an office-based procedure will insure safe, high-quality care tailored to the patient's individual needs. This means that there might be times when a person is not a good candidate to have surgery in a doctor's office. An example is a patient with severe chronic lung disease, or heart disease, or diabetes; these patients might be referred to a hospital or outpatient surgical center, where their specific medical conditions may be managed better. The ASA manual, assembled by the ASA Committee on Ambulatory Surgical Care and the ASA Task Force on Office-Based Anesthesia, titled *Office-Based Anesthesia: Considerations for Anesthesiologists in Setting Up and Maintaining a Safe Office Anesthesia Environment* (2), suggests several factors that should be taken into consideration when deciding whether the patient would be a good candidate for an office-based anesthetic (see Box 7.2). For any anesthesia provider, it is also important to be able to provide to his or her patient a clear explanation of what a particular anesthetic technique entails.

Box 7.2

- Abnormalities of major organ systems and stability and optimization of any medical illness
- Difficult airway
- Previous adverse experience with anesthesia and surgery (such as malignant hyperthermia)
- Current medications and drug allergies
- Time and nature of the last oral intake (NPO status and ASA preprocedural fasting guidelines)
- History of alcohol or substance use or abuse
- Presence of an adult who assumes responsibility specifically for caring for and accompanying the patient from the office

---

MONITORED ANESTHESIA CARE: WHAT DOES THIS REALLY MEAN?

The ASA originally issued its position on MAC in 1986, and it was last amended in 2005. The statement has undergone several revisions over the years (3). The current statement defines MAC as follows:

Monitored anesthesia care is a specific anesthesia service for a diagnostic or therapeutic procedure. Indications for monitored anesthesia care include the nature of the procedure, the patient's clinical condition and / or the potential need to convert to a general or regional anesthetic. Monitored anesthesia care includes all aspects of anesthesia care—a preprocedure visit, intraprocedure care and postprocedure anesthesia management.

During MAC, the anesthesiologist provides or medically directs a number of specific services, including, but not limited to, diagnosis and treatment of clinical problems that occur during the procedure; support of vital functions; administration of sedatives, analgesics, hypnotics, anesthetic agents, or other medications as necessary for patient safety; psychological support and physical comfort; and provision of other medical services as needed to complete the procedure safely. "Monitored anesthesia care may include varying levels of sedation, analgesia, and anxiolysis as necessary." Only qualified personal should administer monitored anesthesia, because "the provider of monitored anesthesia care must be prepared and qualified to convert to general anesthesia when necessary." In an effort to distinguish monitored anesthesia from general anesthesia, in 2003 the ASA added to the statement the following definition:

If the patient loses consciousness and the ability to respond purposefully, the anesthesia care is a general anesthetic, irrespective of whether airway instrumentation is required.

A patient might ask the anesthesia provider to help him or her understand the concept of different levels of sedation, and how they differ from general anesthesia. In 2004, the ASA House of Delegates amended its guidelines on the *Continuum of Depth of Sedation, Definition of General Anesthesia, and Levels of Sedation / Analgesia* (4). According to this document, different levels of sedation are determined based on the patient's responsiveness, the status of the patient's airway, whether the patient is breathing spontaneously or not, and the patient's cardiovascular function (see Table 5.1). Definitions of the depth of sedation were provided and can be found in Chapter 5.

Is there a difference between MAC and conscious sedation? Because there is a variety of individuals who administer sedative medications, the ASA House of Delegates in 2004 issued a statement distinguishing MAC from moderate sedation (what the public recognizes as "conscious sedation") (5). This is based on the different levels of sedation as noted in Table 5.1.

Following is an excerpt from *Distinguishing Monitored Anesthesia Care From Moderate Sedation / Analgesia (Conscious Sedation)*:

Moderate Sedation / Analgesia (Conscious Sedation; hereinafter known as Moderate Sedation) is a physician service recognized in the CPT procedural coding system. During Moderate Sedation, a physician supervises or personally administers sedative and / or analgesic medications that can allay patient anxiety and control pain during a diagnostic or therapeutic procedure. Such drug-induced depression of a patient's level of consciousness to a "moderate" level of sedation, as defined in JCAHO standards, is intended to facilitate the successful performance of the diagnostic or therapeutic procedure while providing patient comfort and cooperation. Physicians providing moderate sedation must be qualified to recognize "deep" sedation, manage its consequences and adjust the level of sedation to a "moderate" or lesser level. The continual assessment of the effects of sedative or analgesic medications on the level of consciousness and on cardiac and respiratory function is an integral element of this service.

Furthermore, the ASA has defined MAC in its *Position on Monitored Anesthesia Care*, last amended in 2005 (3). This physician service can be distinguished from moderate sedation in several ways (see Box 7.3).

Box 7.3

An essential component of MAC is the anesthesia assessment and management of a patient's actual or anticipated physiologic derangements or medical problems that may occur during a diagnostic or therapeutic procedure. While MAC may include the administration of sedatives and/or analgesics often used for moderate sedation, the provider of MAC must be prepared for and qualified to convert to general anesthesia when necessary. Additionally, a provider's ability to intervene to rescue a patient's airway from any sedation-induced compromise is a prerequisite for the qualifications to provide MAC. By contrast, moderate sedation is not expected to induce depths of sedation that would impair the patient's own ability to maintain the integrity of his or her airway. These components of MAC are unique aspects of an anesthesia service that are not part of moderate sedation.

The administration of sedatives, hypnotics, analgesics, as well as anesthetic drugs commonly used for the induction and maintenance of general anesthesia is often, but not always, a part of MAC. In some patients who may require only minimal sedation, MAC is often indicated because even small doses of these medications could precipitate adverse physiologic responses that would necessitate acute clinical interventions and resuscitation. If a patient's condition and/or a procedural requirement is likely to require sedation to a "deep" level or even to a transient period of general anesthesia, only a practitioner privileged to provide anesthesia services should be allowed to manage the sedation. Due to the strong likelihood that "deep" sedation may, with or without intention, transition to general anesthesia, the skills of an anesthesia provider are necessary to manage the effects of general anesthesia on the patient as well as to return the patient quickly to a state of "deep" or lesser sedation.

Like all anesthesia services, MAC includes an array of postprocedure responsibilities beyond the expectations of practitioners providing moderate sedation, including assuring a return to full consciousness, relief of pain, management of adverse physiologic responses or side effects from medications administered during the procedure, as well as the diagnosis and treatment of coexisting medical problems.

MAC allows for the safe administration of a maximal depth of sedation in excess of that provided during moderate sedation. The ability to adjust the sedation level from full consciousness to general anesthesia during the course

> **Box 7.3** *Continued*
> of a procedure provides maximal flexibility in matching sedation level to patient needs and procedural requirements. In situations where the procedure is more invasive or when the patient is especially fragile, optimizing sedation level is necessary to achieve ideal procedural conditions.
>
> *In summary, MAC is a physician service which is clearly distinct from moderate sedation due to the expectations and qualifications of the provider who must be able to utilize all anesthesia resources to support life and to provide patient comfort and safety during a diagnostic or therapeutic procedure.*

WHICH IS THE SAFEST CHOICE?

A patient may often ask his or her anesthesia provider, *"I know about the choices of anesthesia, the different levels of consciousness. Is there any statistical evidence to verify which is the safest choice of anesthesia for me?"* This is a complex question that cannot be answered with a simple "yes" or "no".

Physicians often use the term *"evidence-based medicine"* to substantiate the way they currently practice in their respective fields. Anesthesiologists, just like other practitioners, would like to base many of their clinical decisions on the most current available literature.

Approximately 80% of all surgeries are now being performed on an outpatient basis, and one fourth of these will be performed in an office-based setting. This amounts to approximately 10 million office-based procedures. The growth has been in an exponential pattern over the past decade—twice as many office-based procedures are being performed currently compared with the number in 1995. To provide a basis for evidence-based guidelines regarding safety and the choices of anesthesia while keeping up with the dramatic increase in numbers of patients, large samples of patients are needed when evaluating the current practices. Most of the literature is based on cases performed in the past. This information was obtained from chart reviews and questionnaires sent to a variety of physicians with a variety of credentials (plastic surgeons, oromaxillofacial surgeons, dermatologists). Most of the literature was based on a small sample of patients. To establish a useful guideline, one requires a large sample of patients with similar demographics undergoing the same procedure in different parts of the country, by similar types of surgeons with similar training.

Without having a "gold standard" for a guideline that would specifically point to the "safest" choice of anesthesia, we will present a few recent large-scale studies. We can then make a few general statements about safety in the office-based setting, including the safety of different types of anesthesia. Mentioned in the following text is a list of important articles on safety in OBA, followed by a brief summary of major findings and conclusions (see Box 7.4).

> **Box 7.4**
>
> Bitar G, Mullis W, Jacobs W, et al. Safety and efficacy of office-based surgery with monitored anesthesia care/sedation in 4778 consecutive plastic surgery procedures. *Plast Reconstr Surg.* 2003;111(1):150–156.
>
> Byrd HS, Barton FE, Orenstein HH, et al. Safety and efficacy in an accredited outpatient plastic surgery facility: A review of 5316 consecutive cases. *Plast Reconstr Surg.* 2003;112(2):636–641.
>
> Coldiron B, Shreve E, Balkrishnan R, et al. Patient injuries from surgical procedures performed in medical offices: Three years of Florida data. *Dermatol Surg.* 2004;30(12 Pt 1):1435–1443.

Box 7.4 *Continued*

D'Eramo EM, Bookless SJ, Howard JB, et al. Adverse events with outpatient anesthesia in Massachusetts. *J Oral Maxillofac Surg.* 2003;61(7):793–800.

Hancox JG, Venkat AP, Coldiron B, et al. The safety of office-based surgery: Review of recent literature from several disciplines. *Arch Dermatol.* 2004;140(11):1379–1382.

Hoefflin SM, Bornstein JB, Gordon M, et al. General anesthesia in an office-based plastic surgical facility: A report on more than 23,000 consecutive office-based procedures under general anesthesia with no significant anesthetic complications. *Plast Reconstr Surg.* 2001;107(1):243–257.

Iverson RE. American Society of Plastic Surgeons Task Force on Patient Safety in Office-Based Facilities. Patient safety in office-based surgery facilities: I. Procedures in the office-based surgery setting. *Plast Reconstr Surg.* 2002;110(5):1337–1342.

Morello DC, Colon GA, Fredricks S, et al. Patient safety in accredited office surgical facilities. *Plast Reconstr Surg.* 1997;99(6):1496–1500.

Perrott DH, Yuen JP, Andresen RV, et al. Office-based ambulatory anesthesia: Outcomes of clinical practice of oral and maxillofacial surgeons. *J Oral Maxillofac Surg.* 2003;61(9):983–995.

Vila H, Soto R, Cantor AB, et al. Comparative outcomes analysis of procedures performed in physician offices and ambulatory surgery centers. *Arch Surg.* 2003;138(9):991–995.

Waddle JP, Coleman JE. Discussion of the article by Hoefflin et al. above. *Plast Reconstr Surg.* 2001;107(1):256–258.

Warner MA, Shields SE, Chute CG, et al. Major morbidity and mortality within 1 month of ambulatory surgery and anesthesia. *J Am Med Inform Assoc.* 1993; 270(12):1437–1441.

OFFICE-BASED ANESTHESIA—A REVIEW OF THE MOST RECENT LITERATURE

Performing certain surgical procedures in the office offers many benefits to the patient and the physician. The office-based practice may offer convenience, easy scheduling, added privacy, and decreased expenses. Several studies have looked at adverse events associated with office procedures to determine whether office-based surgical procedures are as safe as those performed in an accredited ambulatory surgical center or an acute care facility (see Table 7.1). Hancox et al. (6), in the review article about the outcomes and mortality of office-based surgery, suggested that if the office-based surgery is as safe as inpatient surgery or surgery in an ambulatory surgicenter (ASC), then the convenience, decreased cost (60%–70%), and ease of scheduling justify the shift from the hospital to the office-based setting. This article reviewed the literature from the general and plastic surgery, medical, health regulatory, and dermatology and summarized the findings. Based on this, the authors concluded that office-based surgery is safe and cost effective, and cautioned against attempts to restrict or prohibit this aspect of medical care.

Morello et al. (7) evaluated adverse events and deaths in 400,675 procedures in 241 plastic surgery offices accredited by the American Association for Accreditation of Ambulatory Surgery Facilities (AAAASF) during a 5-year period. The adverse event rate had an incidence of 0.47%, and there were seven deaths, with a mortality incidence of 0.0017% (<1 in 57,000 procedures). Their conclusion was that the overall risk in an accredited office (i.e., plastic surgical facility) was comparable to that in a freestanding or hospital ambulatory surgical facility. The authors believe that plastic surgery procedures done by a board-certified plastic surgeon in an accredited office facility show an "excellent safety record."

Table 7.1. Review of the most recent literature

Paper	Major Findings
Hoefflin et al.	23,000 procedures under general anesthesia: no deaths or significant complications
Perrott et al.	34,391 patients studied, with 1.3% overall complication rate: local anesthesia: 0.4%; conscious sedation: 0.9%; general anesthesia: 1.5%
D'Eramo et al.	1,706,100 patient retrospective study of oral and maxillofacial procedures: syncope most common complication; 1/853,000 mortality rate
Bitar et al.	4,778 procedures under intravenous sedation: no deaths reported; 12 complications, with PONV being most common
Vila et al.	Relative risk for injury and death for office vs. ambulatory surgery centers: 12.4% and 11.8%, respectively
	Approximately 10-fold increased risk of adverse events and death in office setting
Coldiron et al.	No increased risk of death from office procedures compared with ambulatory surgery procedures

PONV, postoperative nausea and vomiting.

Byrd et al. (8) reviewed 5,316 consecutive cases regarding safety and efficacy in an accredited outpatient plastic surgery facility between 1995–2000 in Dallas Day Surgery Center in Dallas, Texas. They describe the advantages of the office-based setting as having greater control of scheduling, greater privacy for the patient and surgeon, and increased efficiency and consistency in nursing and support personnel. Most cases were cosmetic procedures. During this 6-year period, 35 complications (0.7%) and no deaths were reported. Most of the complications were secondary to hematoma formation. The authors suggested that anesthesia must be delivered by a skilled licensed anesthesia practitioner, and that each case should be individualized based on the magnitude of the operation and the medical condition of the patient. The type of anesthesia and procedure to be performed should involve prior communication between the surgeon and the anesthesia provider. There are no good data available that can exclude a procedure from being performed in an outpatient surgical facility. However, potential blood loss, fluid and electrolyte shifts, postoperative pain, and the extent of anatomic dissection should be considered when choosing the proper facility. A procedure with >500 mL blood loss should be performed where blood products are readily available. The convenience and cost savings of an outpatient surgical facility are ultimately successful if patient safety is preserved.

Iverson (9), together with the American Society of Plastic Surgeons Task Force on Patient Safety in Office-Based Facilities admitted that there is a limited amount of data on patient safety in the office setting. Table 7.2 lists data from the AAAASF census study and two large retrospective studies looking at a private group practice outpatient surgery facility. These studies examined rates of overall complications, incidence of hemorrhage, infection, death, return to the operating room, and the need for hospitalization. These data show that complication rates in office facilities involving plastic surgery procedures appear to be very low.

Hoefflin et al. (10) in an effort to validate the safety of general anesthesia, reported on 23,000 consecutive cases over an 18-year period. Their report is

Table 7.2.   Data from the American Association for Accreditation of Ambulatory Surgery Facilities' census study and two large retrospective studies looking at a private group practice outpatient surgery facility

No. of Cases (%)	Office-Based Safety and Plastic Surgery		
	Morello et al. 400,675	Byrd et al. 5,316	Rose et al. 5,734
Complications	0.47	0.6	0.12
Hemorrhage	0.24	0.46	0.79
Infection	0.09	0.11	0.02
Death	0.0017	0	0
Return to OR	0.15	0.66	0.79
Hospitalization	0.03	0.13	0.12

From: Iverson RE. American Society of Plastic Surgeons Task Force on Patient Safety in Office-Based Facilities. Patient safety in office-based surgery facilities: I. Procedures in the office-based surgery setting. *Plast Reconstr Surg.* 2002;110(5):1337–1342.

a detailed account of the policies and procedures in which general anesthesia was used in all patients, with no deaths and no significant complications. According to the authors, the advantages of general anesthesia over intravenous sedation include (a) better control of the airway, (b) the surgeon's ability to focus on the procedure rather than monitor the level of anesthesia, and (c) elimination of variability in the level of consciousness seen with intravenous sedation. Overall, the general anesthesia protocol presented in the article uniformly provided a high degree of safety, comfort, and pleasant experience for the patient, surgeon, and the anesthesia provider. Part of this positive experience for the patient is an adequate preoperative evaluation, along with education about what to expect from the anesthesia and surgery. A patient who is well informed is less anxious, requires less anesthesia, and recovers more rapidly. It also emphasizes the fact that the experience does not end until the patient is healed. The process is a continuum, from the preoperative period to the postoperative period—not simply while the patient is in the operating room. While the authors state that office-based surgery is cost effective for the patient, they also emphasize the importance of individualizing patient treatment, controlling the overall environment, and providing a more comfortable, caring, and more private setting than is available at most hospitals. At a well-run office-based facility there may be a greater indulgence in the patient because the staff is more trained and oriented to this type of specialty care. It is noted that none of this would be important unless the office-based facility were as safe as seen in a freestanding ambulatory surgical center or an acute care hospital.

Waddle and Coleman (11), in discussing the Hoefflin et al. (10) article, states that many surgeons and anesthesia personnel use intravenous sedation instead of general anesthesia because they believe that general anesthesia is riskier. On a statistical basis, there is somewhat of a bias when comparing the two types of anesthesia because those procedures that require general anesthesia are often longer, more complicated, and associated with more blood loss and pain than those procedures that require intravenous sedation. To find out whether this is actually true requires a large sample size. Studies of this nature are time consuming and labor intensive, which makes them prohibitive. The incidence of morbidity and mortality after ambulatory surgery is low.

Warner et al. (12) performed a 30-day follow-up study of 38,598 ambulatory patients to determine the incidence and time sequence of mortality and major morbidity following surgery. They found four deaths, two from myocardial infarctions and two from automobile accidents. The rate of major morbidity was 0.08% (stroke, myocardial infarction, pulmonary embolism, respiratory failure). More than one third of the major morbidity occurred 48 hours or later following discharge. Minor morbidity of general anesthesia included nausea and vomiting (4.7%), dental damage (0.02%), corneal abrasion (0.056%), sore throat (28%), nerve injury (0.47%), and shivering (2.2%). The authors concluded that the overall morbidity and mortality rates were very low.

Perrott et al. (13) evaluated 34,391 patients undergoing oral and maxillofacial surgery in the office-based setting during a 1-year period in 2001. Of these, 71.9% received deep sedation/general anesthesia, 15.5% received conscious sedation, and the rest received local anesthesia. The overall complication rate was 1.3%, and described as "minor and self-limiting." By examining data by anesthesia type, it appears that the complication rates were 0.4% with local anesthesia, 0.9% with conscious sedation and 1.5% with general anesthesia. The study results were based on the largest prospective patient study sample ever enrolled while evaluating the office-based setting. The patient satisfaction was extremely high with 95% of patients recommending the anesthetic technique to another loved one. The authors concluded that the administration of deep sedation, general anesthesia, conscious sedation, or local anesthesia by oral and maxillofacial surgeon teams was safe.

D'Eramo et al. (14) conducted a retrospective practitioner survey to evaluate adverse events associated with outpatient anesthesia in 1.7 million patients in Massachusetts treated between 1995 and 1999. It was largely based on a questionnaire mailed to 157 practicing oral and maxillofacial surgeons. The most common event was syncope ("passing out" presumably due to a vasovagal phenomenon) present in 1 in 160 cases with local anesthesia. Two treatment-related deaths were recorded during this period, making the overall dental anesthesia mortality rate of 1 per 835,000.

Some studies specifically looked at the safety of MAC and intravenous sedation in the office. For example, Bitar et al. (15) reviewed medical records of 3,615 consecutive patients who had undergone 4,778 plastic surgery procedures over a 1-year period (1999–2000). All procedures were performed by board-certified plastic surgeons and board-certified anesthesia personnel. The study found no deaths, ventilator requirements, deep venous thrombosis, or pulmonary emboli. There were 12 anesthetic complications, including nausea and vomiting (most common), dyspnea, one emergent intubation, and two unplanned hospital admissions.

One the other hand, some studies have questioned the safety of office-based surgery and produced data that contradicts others' conclusions that office is as safe as an ambulatory surgical center or a hospital facility. One controversial study by Vila et al. (16), "*Comparative Outcomes Analysis of Procedures Performed in Physician Offices and Ambulatory Surgery Centers,*" compared patient safety in an ambulatory surgical center with that in an office setting. The authors examined adverse incident reports presented to the Florida Board of Medicine between 2000 and 2002. After close examination of the data, the authors found that adverse incidents occurred at a rate of 66 and 5.3 per 100,000 procedures in offices and ambulatory surgical centers, respectively. The death rate per 100,000 procedures was found to be 9.2 in the offices and only 0.78 in ambulatory surgery centers. Analyzing these data further, the authors found that the relative risks for injuries and deaths for office procedures versus ambulatory surgery centers were 12.4 and 11.8, respectively. They concluded that if all office procedures had been performed in ambulatory surgery centers, approximately 43 injuries and 6 deaths per year could have been prevented.

In response to the Vila et al. (16) study, Coldiron et al. (17) refuted some of the study's findings. This paper evaluated surgical incidents in office-based settings using 3 years of Florida data from 2000 to 2003. The latter found several flaws in the way the Vila et al. study was conducted, claiming that it excluded in its analysis the credentials of the surgeon, office accreditation, and the presence or absence of an anesthesiologist or certified registered nurse anesthetist during the case. Coldiron et al. found little evidence, based on the data available, that the presence of an anesthesiologist and mandating office accreditation would have any "beneficial impact" on the safety of office-based surgery. The "primary flaw" of the Vila et al. article, Coldiron et al. claim, is the measurement error bias in the calculation of office deaths estimates. In calculating office death rates compared with ambulatory surgery centers, Vila et al. used all reported deaths in the offices for the numerator, but the denominator contained only procedure estimates from registered office settings—this would lead to an overestimate of the relative death risk in the office. Also, in its relative risk calculations for office-based procedures, Vila et al. combined both accredited and nonaccredited facilities, and also some of the deaths occurred after the patient was discharged. Therefore, Coldiron et al. concluded that the apparently increased relative risk of death in the office was due less to the location of the surgery but more to general anesthesia being performed in the office (this statement is contradicted by Hoefflin et al. who reported no deaths in 23,000 procedures performed under general anesthesia (10). Finally, Coldiron et al. claimed that a) Vila excluded credentials of the surgeon, office accreditation, and presence or absence of an anesthesiologist or certified nurse anesthetist during the case, and that b) it seemed to make little difference in outcome, "negating Vila's conclusions that the presence of an anesthesiologist during all office procedures and mandating office accreditation would have beneficial impact." The addendum to the last statement from Caldiron et al. should be procedures—the added risk due to general anesthesia being performed, not due to the location of the procedure.

Finally, Hancox et al. (6) reviewed recent literature, specifically addressing adverse outcomes and mortality of office-based surgical procedures. Despite all the conflicting reports regarding the safety of office-based surgery, adverse event reporting should be uniform in order for large scale studies to correctly assess the risk. Until this is done, no definitive conclusions can be drawn, and opinion may be swayed by anecdotes and sensationalism in the media. The authors conclude with the following statement, which is a fair conclusion based on the currently available evidence:

We believe that office-based surgery should only be performed by properly trained physicians working within their scope of practice. We also acknowledge that, in selected cases, certified anesthetists or anesthesiologists should administer anesthesia and carefully monitor patients. We also advocate the uniform reporting of adverse events and mortality related to office-based surgery, so that the proper analysis can be performed and patient safety can be assured. With the available data, and in absence of the gold standard of randomized prospective trials, we contend that office-based surgery is safe and cost-effective (6).

Without doubt, more studies need to be done to determine what the best practices might be as we are faced with the exponential growth of office-based surgery. The ASA, many states, and other professional societies have created their own guidelines that attempt to standardize office-based practice.

In summary, there are no "simple" questions and no "easy" answers. There is also conflicting data regarding the safety of office-based surgery compared with surgery performed in ambulatory surgical centers and acute care hospitals. However, most authorities would agree that a safe OBA practice calls for:

An educated, capable provider working in an accredited facility with policies governing patient selection and healthcare personnel.

The realities of the current health care environment dictate that office-based surgery will continue to grow and be popular with both patients and physicians. Based on this, it is imperative for our profession to promote specific practice guidelines, proper provider training, facility accreditation, and appropriate patient and procedure selection.

REFERENCES

1. American Society of Anesthesiologists. *Guidelines for office-based anesthesia.* (Approved by ASA House of Delegates in 1999, and last affirmed on October 27, 2004). ASA House of Delegates; Available at: http://www.asahq.org/publicationsandServices/standards/12.pdf. 2004.
2. American Society of Anesthesiologists. *Office-based anesthesia: Considerations for anesthesiologists in setting up and maintaining a safe office anesthesia environment (ASA Committee on Ambulatory Surgical Care and ASA Task Force on Office-Based Anesthesia.* Available at: http://www.asahq.org/publicationsAndServices/office.pdf. 2002.
3. American Society of Anesthesiologists. *Position on monitored anesthesia care.* (Approved by House of Delegates on October 21, 1986, amended on October 25, 2005). ASA House of Delegates; Available at: www.asahq.org/publicationsAndServices/standards/23.pdf. 2005.
4. American Society of Anesthesiologists. *Continuum of depth of sedation. Definition of general anesthesia and levels of sedation/analgesia.* (Approved by ASA House of Delegates on October 13, 1999, and amended on October 27, 2004). ASA House of Delegates; Available at: http://www.asahq.org/publicationsAndServices/standards/20.pdf. 2004.
5. American Society of Anesthesiologists. *Distinguishing monitored anesthesia care ("MAC") from moderate sedation/analgesia-conscious sedation.* (Approved by the ASA House of Delegates on October 27, 2004). ASA House of Delegates; Available at: www.asahq.org/publicationsAndServices/standards/35.pdf. 2004.
6. Hancox JG, Venkat A, Coldiron B, et al. The safety of office-based surgery: Review of recent literature form several disciplines. *Arch Dermatol.* 2004; 140(11):1379–1382.
7. Morello DC, Colon GA, Fredricks S, et al. Patient safety in accredited office surgical facilities. *Plast Reconstr Surg.* 1997;99(6):1496–1500.
8. Byrd HS, Barton FE, Orenstein HH, et al. Safety and efficacy in an accredited outpatient plastic surgery facility: A review of 5316 consecutive cases. *Plast Reconstr Surg.* 2003;112(2):636–641.
9. Iverson RE. American Society of Plastic Surgeons Task Force on Patient Safety in Office-Based Facilities. Patient safety in office-based surgery facilities: I. Procedures in the office-based surgery setting. *Plast Reconstr Surg.* 2002;110(5):1337–1342.
10. Hoefflin SM, Bornstein JB, Gordon M, et al. General anesthesia in an office-based plastic surgical facility: A report on more than 23,000 consecutive office-based procedures under general anesthesia with no significant anesthetic complications. *Plast Reconstr Surg.* 2001;107(1):243–257.
11. Waddle JP, Coleman JE. Discussion of the article by Hoefflin et al. above. *Plast Reconstr Surg.* 2001;107(1):256–258.
12. Warner M, Chute C. Major morbidity and mortality within 1 month of ambulatory surgery and anesthesia. *JAMA.* 1993;270:1437.

13. Perrott DH, Yuen JP, Andresen RV, et al. Office-based ambulatory anesthesia: Outcomes of clinical practice of oral and maxillofacial surgeons. *J Oral Maxillofac Surg*. 2003;61(9):983–995.
14. D'Eramo EM, Bookless SJ, Howard JB, et al. Adverse events with outpatient anesthesia in Massachusetts. *J Oral Maxillofac Surg*. 2003;61(983):95.
15. Bitar G, Mullis W, Jacobs W, et al. Safety and efficacy of office-based surgery with monitored anesthesia care/sedation in 4778 consecutive plastic surgery procedures. *Plast Reconstr Surg*. 2003;111(1):150–156.
16. Vila H, Soto R, Cantor AB, et al. Comparative outcomes analysis of procedures performed in physician offices and ambulatory surgery centers. *Arch Surg*. 2003;138(9):991–995.
17. Coldiron B, Shreve E, Balkrishnan R, et al. Patient injuries from surgical procedures performed in medical offices: Three years of Florida data. *Dermatol Surg*. 2004;30((12 Pt 1)):1435–1443.

Closed Claims Project

Karinne M. Jervis, Richard D. Urman, and Fred E. Shapiro

The Closed Claims Project, established in 1984 by the American Society of Anesthesiologists (ASA), was formed to recognize and formulate procedures to prevent anesthesia-related complications. The driving force behind this study was the dichotomy between the number of anesthesiologists and the amount of malpractice claims. At that time anesthesiologists comprised only 3% of the population of physicians; however they accounted for 11% of the total malpractice claims—an inordinate amount compared with the number of physicians. The ASA Closed Claims Project is conducted by the ASA Committee on Profession Liability. This committee comprised 35 insurance companies and anesthesiology reviewers that review closed claims that were anesthesiology-related. The information and statistics provided by the Closed Claims Project has influenced the practice of anesthesia and stimulated research in multiple areas—especially in the burgeoning areas of office-based anesthesia. Owing to the identification of adverse effects complied with in the 30-year review, the practice of anesthesia has become safer since the inception of the Closed Claims Project, and further extrapolation of data from 3 decades of research to the new area of office-based anesthesia will make this uncharted and under-investigated area of anesthesia safer as well.

LESSONS LEARNED FROM THE STUDY

The compilation of data has demonstrated that most of the claims have occurred with the following:

- Healthy adults undergoing elective procedures
- Women (59% of claims)
- Adults (91% of claims)
- ASA 1 or 2 (69% of claims)

Lessons learned from the study demonstrated the need for further monitoring of patients under anesthesia. After the implementation of further monitoring, pulse oximetry, and end-tidal capnography, the rate of preventable anesthetic complications, if further monitoring had been employed, decreased from 39% of claims in the 1970s to 9% in the 1990s (1,2).

HOW DOES THIS INFORMATION PERTAIN TO OFFICE-BASED ANESTHESIA?

To date, there have only been a few claims from the office-based anesthesia setting, but there are some startling and interesting comparisons between the Closed Claims Project data of the 1980s and the early 2000s (see Table 8.1 and Figure 8.1). If you believe in the philosophy that "history repeats itself," this is an excellent example (3). Interestingly, the demographics of the following claims are similar:

- Middle-aged women
- ASA 1 or 2
- Elective surgery
- General anesthesia

Adverse events included the following:

- Airway obstruction (bronchospasm/laryngospasm)
- Inadequate ventilatory support
- Drug errors

Table 8.1. Comparisons between the Closed Claims Project data of the 1980s and the early 2000s

	Ambulatory Anesthesia ($n = 753$)	Office-Based Anesthesia ($n = 14$)
Age (mean in years)	41	45
Female (%)	58	64
ASA 1–2 (%)	82	89
Elective surgery (%)	97	100
Anesthesia type		
General (%)	66	71
MAC (%)	10	14
Surgical procedure		
Dental (%)	3	21
Plastic surgery (%)	32[a]	21[a]
Other (%)	64[b]	14[b]

[a]$p < 0.05$ Ambulatory vs. Office-Based Anesthesia
[b]$p < 0.01$ Ambulatory vs. Office-Based Anesthesia
Percentages do not equal 100% due to rounding
MAC, monitored anesthesia care.

Box 8.1

The Conclusion
"All the potentially preventable office-based injuries resulted from adverse respiratory events in the recovery or postoperative periods, which were judged to be preventable by use of pulse oximetry (2)."

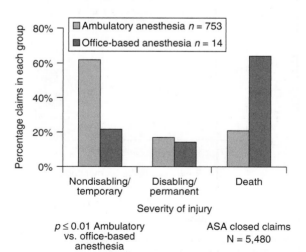

Figure 8.1. Severity of injury in ambulatory anesthesia versus office-based claims. ASA, American Society of Anesthesiologists.
American Society of Anesthesiologists. *Newsletter.* 2001;65(6):7.

SAFETY CONCERNS

Acknowledging this data, it becomes necessary to review whether requiring patients to remain observed by the anesthesiologist for direct monitoring will have better outcomes. Is the practice of ambulatory anesthesia in an office-based setting truly safe? For many patients, the idea of having procedures and anesthesia in an office-based setting is a means to reduce anxiety, improve patient satisfaction, and increase patient convenience. There is concern that the immense expansion of office-based anesthesia cases has occurred without the recognition of patient safety (4). Several office-based surgical settings have adapted to the need to monitor patients for prolonged periods—settings where patients are not only pampered after surgery but are monitored for periods of respiratory or cardiac demise. With an increasingly litigious society and with the need to provide better care for patients, a look back to the past of prolonged hospital stays and better monitoring may again become the norm.

The anesthesiologist in an office-based setting must therefore take on the role as the true perioperative physician in order to assume and ensure that the patient's safety is paramount. With the increasing numbers of office-based settings, office-based surgery has provided this opportunity of embellishing this diverse role (5). To establish a setting of safety, the office setting should be held at standards similar to that of a hospital or even an ambulatory surgical setting. In this respect, the anesthesiologist must therefore become the patient's advocate—advocating for the procurement of resuscitation materials, emergency protocols, preassessment strategies, and postoperative recovery monitoring. By establishing criteria to ensure patient safety, pre-, intra-, and postoperatively, anesthesiologists will secure an even more important role in the office-based setting (see Figure 8.2).

In a recent paper, Bhananker et al. (6) performed a closed claims analysis of the injuries associated with monitored anesthesia care (MAC). These data

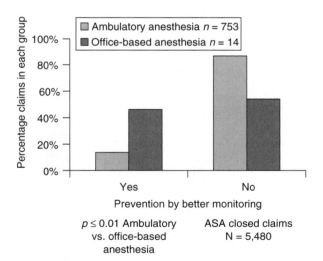

Figure 8.2.   Prevention of injury in ambulatory anesthesia versus office-based claims. ASA, American Society of Anesthesiologists.
American Society of Anesthesiologists. *Newsletter.* 2001;65(6):7.

Table 8.2. Analysis of the injuries associated with monitored anesthesia care

Mechanisms of Injury	MAC (N = 121) n (%)	GA (N = 1,519) n (%)	RA (N = 312) n (%)
Respiratory event	29 (24)	337 (22)	11 (4)
Inadequate oxygenation/ventilation	22 (18)	33 (2)	5 (2)
Cardiovascular event	17 (14)	253 (17)	23 (7)
Equipment failure/malfunction	25 (21)	199 (13)	8 (3)
Cautery fires	20 (17)	10 (1)	1 (0)
Related to regional block	2 (2)	7 (0)	168 (54)
Inadequate anesthesia/patient movement	13 (11)	42 (3)	7 (2)
Medication related	11 (9)	95 (6)	11 (4)
Other events[a]	24 (20)	586 (39)	84 (27)

[a] Includes surgical technique/patient condition, patient fell, operation/location, positioning, failure to diagnose, other known damages, no damaging event, and unknown.
MAC, monitored anesthesia care; GA, general anesthesia; RA, regional anesthesia.
From: Bhananker SM, Posner KL, Cheney FW, et al. Injury and liability associated with monitored anesthesia care: A closed claims analysis. *Anesthesiology.* 2006;104(2):228–234.

refer to procedures performed in all kinds of health care settings, such as offices, ambulatory surgicenters, and acute care hospitals. The authors examined closed malpractice claims in the ASA Closed Claims Database since 1990. The authors found that more than 40% of claims associated with MAC involved death or permanent brain damage similar to general anesthesia claims, and that respiratory depression was the most common mechanism of injury (21%). They concluded that almost half (46%) of the claims could have been prevented by the following:

- Better monitoring, including capnography
- Improved vigilance
- Audible alarms

In addition, the use of electrocautery in the presence of a nearby supplemental oxygen source during facial surgery resulted in 17% of the claims. Other mechanisms of injury included cardiovascular events, equipment failure and malfunction, injuries related to regional blocks and inadequate anesthesia, and medication errors. Table 8.2 summarizes this paper's major findings.

On the basis of these and other data, we must think "outside-the-box" and look at other ways to improve safety in the operating room. Carefully designed medical simulation exercises addressing common issues encountered in an office-based practice would be one such option. Indeed, looking at the statistics presented by various closed claims and other outcomes studies, one can create a useful simulation and crisis management curriculum addressing most common causes of patient morbidity and mortality in ambulatory and office-based settings.

MEDICAL SIMULATION IN THE OFFICE SETTING

The use of medical simulation has become an important tool in medicine. It has grown significantly over the last decade, and has been used successfully in the aviation industry and the military. The purpose of a simulation exercise is to achieve the following:

- Teach crisis resource management skills
- Help the participant function as a member of the team
- Increase medical knowledge
- Improve clinical and decision-making skills

A simulation exercise allows the participant to review his or her performance and receive constructive feedback. From a patient safety perspective, this can be an invaluable tool to learn and experiment in a risk-free environment. Many hospitals encourage or even mandate that its health care staff regularly participate in the simulator program, and some malpractice insurers even offer premium discounts after the successful completion of such a course.

Simulation exercises can be created for all levels of training and for all types of practitioners, making it a useful experience for a student, a physician-in-training, or a seasoned health care professional. Many major health care facilities offer some kind of simulator training. Many believe that simulation improves learning and performance, and could even lead to fewer medical errors and better patient outcomes. Although such data may be difficult to obtain, simulation exercises generally receive excellent feedback from the participants and have become an integral component of health provider education.

Office-based staff can benefit from simulation training that addresses unique aspects of the office-based practice. The staff should be introduced to the basic principles of event management (7), such as the following:

- Role clarity
- Communication
- Resource management
- Support of team members
- Global assessment techniques

Team training would be critical because offices are often freestanding facilities, and resources and personnel are generally limited. Such team training should involve the *entire* office-based team, including the surgeon, anesthesia provider, and nursing and support staff.

Scenarios can be designed to address the following:

- *Role assignments*
- *Team leadership*
- *Two-way communication*
- *Proper equipment use*
- *Team member support*
- *Situational awareness*

The debriefing session that often follows the actual simulation exercise is just as important. It allows participants to share their experiences and feelings, and assess their performance. They can then decide what went well, and what they could have done differently. The debriefing session often includes the viewing of the recording of the simulation session, and can be quite revealing for the participant.

On the basis of the data given in the preceding text, it is possible to design individual scenarios addressing most common adverse events in the hope of preventing similar future incidents. A particular simulation scenario may involve one or more of the emergencies in Box 8.2.

> ## Box 8.2
>
> **Respiratory:** Loss of airway, pulmonary embolism, pneumothorax, aspiration
> **Cardiovascular:** Myocardial infarction, cardiac arrhythmias, malignant hyperthermia
> **Equipment:** Oxygen failure, machine malfunction
> **Fire:** Fires involving patient or equipment
> **Medication error:** Wrong medication, medication overdose
> **Code Status:** Unknown code status, advanced cardiac life support (ACLS) protocol

The scenarios should stress important aspects of the office-based anesthesia practice, including, but not limited to, the following:

- *Preoperative evaluation*
- *Patient selection*
- *Adverse intraoperative events*
- *Postoperative issues*

The topics mentioned earlier are just a suggestion. Regardless of the scenario, simulation may offer a realistic "on demand" education for all levels of training and expertise. The goal is patient safety and making the staff more confident in providing clinical care and working together as a team.

REFERENCES

1. Cooper P. Behind the scenes at the ASA closed claims project. *ASA Newsl.* 1999;63(6):10–11; http://www.asahq.org/Newsletters/1999/06_99/Behind_0699.html.
2. Lee LA, Domino KB. The closed claims project: Has it influenced anesthetic practice and outcome? *Anesthesiol Clin North Am.* 2002;20(3):485–501.
3. Twersky, et al. Practice options: Considerations in setting up an office-based anesthesia practice. *ASA Newsl.* 1997;61(9):30–32; http://www.asahq.org/Newsletters/1997/09_97/PractOpt_0997.html.
4. Domino K. Office-based anesthesia: Lessons learned from the closed claims project. *ASA Newsl.* 2001;65(6):9–11; http://www.asahq.org/Newsletters/2001/06_01/June01.pdf.
5. Stoelting RK. Office-based anesthesia growth provokes safety fears. *Anesthesia Patient Safety Foundation Newsl.* 2000;15(1):1; http://www.apsf.org/resource_center/newsletter/2000/spring/01-intro.htm.
6. Bhananker SM, Posner KL, Cheney FW, et al.. Injury and liability associated with monitored anesthesia care: A closed claims analysis. *Anesthesiology.* 2006;104(2):228–234.
7. Fish K, Howard S. *Crisis management in anesthesiology.* Philadelphia: Churchill Livingstone; 1994.

Choosing Anesthetic Agents. Which One?

Richard D. Urman and Fred E. Shapiro

A wide variety of anesthetic techniques and agents may be utilized for a given surgical procedure in the hospital-based operating room (OR) setting. However, the office-based OR is unique because of the types of procedures, patient population, anesthetic techniques, and resources employed. This chapter outlines information and practice guidelines that will allow office-based anesthesiology personnel to choose the anesthetic agents and techniques best suited for the procedure being performed. This is critical, in order to ensure that each patient has a safe, pleasant, and comfortable surgical experience.

THE BASICS OF CHOOSING ANESTHETIC AGENTS

The anesthesiologist must choose drugs that fulfill procedure and patient requirements, and facilitate safe and effective administration of anesthesia. This knowledge must be coordinated with the patient's medical history, in order to formulate an optimal plan for the anesthesia care.

There are at least five basic aspects of anesthesia that should be considered for each patient undergoing surgery in the office (see Box 9.1).

Box 9.1

1. Anxiolysis
2. Amnesia
3. Sedation
4. Analgesia
5. Avoidance of side effects
   (i.e., headache, nausea, vomiting, dizziness, drowsiness, and pain)

To meet these requirements, drugs must be chosen that facilitate the administration of anesthesia (see Box 9.2). Because there is no single drug or agent that satisfies all of these requirements and characteristics, several different classes of drugs with different profiles must be utilized in combination to achieve these effects.

Box 9.2 • Drug Characteristics that Facilitate the Administration of Anesthesia

1. Rapid onset
2. Easily controlled depth of sedation
3. Rapid recovery
4. Minimal respiratory effect
5. Cardiovascular stability
6. Nonallergic
7. Minimal active metabolic byproducts

The next step is to assess each patient individually and review his or her medical history, in order to select appropriate drugs and minimize side effects and dangerous drug interactions (see Box 9.3).

Box 9.3

Patient-Specific Factors to Consider Include the Following:
1. Pre-existing medical conditions
2. Drug allergies
3. Patient medications (include herbs and dietary supplements)
4. Social history (e.g., smoking, alcohol, and recreational drug use)
5. Review old medical records, if available

If the patient has previously undergone surgery, it is prudent to look at the old records, noting both the positive and negative experiences, so that the most appropriate perioperative plan may be formulated.

ANESTHETIC TECHNIQUES

Once the anesthesiologist is familiar with the requirements of anesthesia, the characteristics of drugs that facilitate the administration of anesthesia, and the patient's medical history, an anesthetic plan may be further tailored to each patient by choosing an anesthetic technique. Fast-track anesthesia and monitored anesthesia care (MAC) are the two techniques often employed in the office-based OR.

Fast-track anesthesia refers to the art and science of swiftly moving patients into the OR, out of the OR, through the postanesthesia care unit (PACU), and then discharging them home in a relatively short time. This is the true definition of "outpatient surgery." It evolved out of the need for a cost-effective measure to accommodate an increasing number of patients undergoing minimally invasive surgical procedures. The development of short-acting anesthetics, improved methods of pain control, new anesthetic monitoring, more advanced technology devices, and new recovery protocols have facilitated this process. Because of their rapid onset, peak effect, and metabolism, ultra short-acting induction agents and narcotics allow patients to have their procedure with the requirements discussed in the preceding text, awaken in a clear-headed manner, recover quickly, and be discharged home in a relatively short time.

The use of MAC is rapidly gaining acceptance and popularity in plastic surgery. This is due to increasing experience and small modifications of surgical technique and local anesthesia. Currently, a variety of aesthetic procedures are being performed combining a local anesthetic with some form of intravenous sedation. These include breast augmentation and reduction, mastopexy, abdominoplasty, rhytidectomy, rhinoplasty, blepharoplasty, and liposuction.

Before any type of sedation is considered, the anesthesiologist must first evaluate the patient to determine whether the patient is a good candidate for this type of anesthesia. Second, the anesthesiologist must be familiar with the medications used for intravenous sedation and must realize that every patient acts differently with respect to drugs. For instance, "light" sedation for one person might be "deep" sedation for another. Patient safety is of primary concern to any person administering intravenous sedation. The essentials include proper patient selection, careful management of each case by skilled personnel, appropriate drug selection and administration, and adequate continuous monitoring during and after surgery.

The American Society of Anesthesiologists (ASA) has provided guidelines for the safe use of conscious sedation for anesthesiologists and nonanesthesiologists, as outlined in Chapter 5. The obvious benefits of conscious sedation versus general anesthesia include avoidance of the cardiopulmonary effects of general anesthesia, airway injury, postoperative nausea and vomiting (PONV), and positional nerve injuries. The risk of developing deep vein thrombophlebitis as a result of blood pooling in the lower extremities during general anesthesia is also lessened. Refer to the ASA's definition and discussion of MAC in Chapter 5.

ANESTHETIC AGENTS

The discussion in the subsequent text focuses on different classes of drugs currently used in anesthesia. The goal is to provide the office-based anesthesiology personnel with all the necessary information, in order to plan the correct "pharmacologic cocktail" that will guarantee the patient a safe, pleasant, and comfortable experience. Table 9.1 summarizes the most commonly used drug classes and their effects on sedation, anxiolysis, pain, and cardiovascular and respiratory systems. A more extensive discussion of each drug class, with specific emphasis on office-based anesthesia follows.

Local Anesthetics

Local anesthetics can be administered by local infiltration within the area of the wound, through topical administration, or through a peripheral nerve block. The instillation of local anesthetic may reduce the amount of perioperative opioid use, thereby reducing unfavorable side effects. There are obvious advantages of minimizing opioid use, so that patients are able to remain alert, maintain gastrointestinal (GI) function, and improve their ability to ambulate. Dosing is specific to each type of local anesthetic and is based on the patient's weight. Dosages beyond the specified amount for each drug may result in toxicity, leading to mental status changes, seizures, cardiac arrhythmias, and death. Table 9.2 lists the most commonly used local anesthetics, their onset, duration of action, and maximum doses.

Local anesthetics of choice in ambulatory anesthesia include lidocaine, bupivacaine, ropivacaine, and levobupivacaine. Lidocaine has a relatively short duration of action. Bupivacaine has a longer duration of action and a very small therapeutic window. It is associated with profound cardiovascular (arrhythmias, cardiac arrest) and central nervous system (CNS) effects (seizures, CNS depression) in cases of unintentional intravascular injection or overdose. Two new local anesthetic agents, ropivacaine and levobupivacaine, have a greater safety profile with respect to cardiovascular and CNS toxicity. Therefore, these drugs may be safer alternatives to bupivacaine

Table 9.1.   Commonly used drug classes and their effects

Drug Class	Effects				
	Sedation	Anxiolysis	Pain	Cardio-vascular	Respiratory
Local anesthetics	0	0	+	++	+
Barbiturates	++	+	0	+	++
Benzodiazepines	++	++	0	+	++
Ketamine	++	+	++	+	0
Propofol	++	+	0	++	++
Inhalational agents	++	+	++	++	+
α_2 Agonists	++	+	++	+	0
Opioids	++	+	0	+	++

Table 9.2. Commonly used local anesthetics with dosage, onset, and duration of action

Local Anesthetic	Onset	Duration (min)	Maximum Single Dose (mg)
Lidocaine	Rapid	60–120	300
Mepivacaine	Slow	90–180	300
Prilocaine	Slow	60–120	400
Bupivacaine	Slow	240–480	175
Ropivacaine	Slow	240–480	200
Levobupivacaine	Slow	240–480	175
Procaine	Rapid	45–60	500
Chloroprocaine	Rapid	30–45	600
Tetracaine	Slow	60–180	100

From: Stoelting R, Miller R. *Basics of Anesthesia*, 4th ed. Churchill Livingstone, 2000.

for extending the duration of local anesthetic into the postoperative period. In addition, ropivacaine may be a good alternative with a shorter and less intense motor block than bupivacaine (1).

Infiltration of local anesthetic may be performed for small- to moderate-sized and relatively superficial procedures. Lidocaine 0.5% to 1.0% or bupivacaine 0.25% are most commonly used. The addition of epinephrine, a vasoconstrictor that delays absorption of the local anesthetic, in a 1:200,000 dilution (epi = 5 μg/mL) will prolong the duration of action. Bupivacaine 0.25%, ropivacaine 0.25% to 0.5%, or levobupivacaine 0.25% will produce up to 4 hours of pain relief. Surgical site infiltration, in combination with nonopioid analgesics such as acetaminophen or celecoxib may be adequate analgesia for minor surgical procedures and can be used as the basal analgesic technique for all surgical procedures (1).

Midazolam

Midazolam is a rapid, short-acting benzodiazepine that causes profound anxiolysis, amnesia, and sedation. Benzodiazepines act within the CNS to enhance the inhibitory tone of γ-aminobutyric acid (GABA) receptors. Because binding is specific, benzodiazepines have minimal cardiovascular depressant effects in doses used for sedation. Benzodiazepines cause a depression in the ventilatory response curve to CO_2 (a decrease in the slope of the curve). This can become significant when combined with other respiratory depressants.

If midazolam is to be used alone for MAC, the intravenous dose can generally range from 2.5 to 7.5 mg. If used for anxiolysis before induction of general anesthesia, a propofol infusion, or a remifentanil infusion, the typical intravenous dose of midazolam is 1 to 2 mg (2). The infusion rate of midazolam for MAC anesthesia is 1 to 2 μg/kg/min. Midazolam's elimination half-life is approximately 2 hours (3). It is also important to note that there is a marked decrease in midazolam requirements as patients age. Complete recovery after a single dose of 0.1 μg/kg requires approximately 90 minutes. This is the main reason why midazolam is generally not used to induce or maintain loss of consciousness. It is most commonly used as a premedication or for conscious sedation.

Ketamine

Ketamine is a phencyclidine (PCP) derivative that produces a dissociative state, which is accompanied by amnesia and profound analgesia. The patient appears conscious but is unable to process or respond to sensory input. Its mode of action is not well defined, but the mechanism of action is thought to be through N-methyl-D-aspartate (NMDA) receptor antagonism. In contrast to other anesthetic agents, ketamine stimulates the sympathetic nervous system to increase heart rate (HR), systemic blood pressure (BP), and pulmonary artery BP. Ketamine can therefore be used to balance the negative cardiovascular effects of propofol. Owing to its effects on the sympathetic nervous system, ketamine should be avoided in patients with the following:

1. Coronary artery disease
2. Uncontrolled hypertension
3. Congestive heart failure
4. Arterial aneurysms

Respiratory depressant effects of ketamine are minimal, upper airway reflexes remain largely intact, and the sympathomimetic effect may alleviate bronchospasm. Ketamine does increase salivation, which can be attenuated by premedication with an anticholinergic agent. Ketamine also increases cerebral oxygen consumption, cerebral blood flow, and intracranial pressure. It should therefore be avoided in patients with space occupying intracranial lesions, head trauma, or intracranial hypertension. The induction dose of ketamine is 1 to 2 mg per kg IV and 3 to 4 mg IM. The intravenous sedative dose is in the range of 5 to 15 μg/kg/min and must be titrated to effect (2). The elimination half-life is 2 to 4 hours. Ketamine is associated with a high incidence of psychomimetic effects. Restlessness and agitation may occur on emergence, and hallucinations and unpleasant dreams may occur postoperatively. Patients at higher risk for psychomimetic effects include females, older age, and patients receiving doses >2 mg per kg. These effects can be greatly reduced by the concurrent use of propofol and midazolam (4,5) (see Tables 9.3 and 9.4).

Table 9.3. Examples of dosing regimens for various anesthetic intravenous agents during general anesthesia in the ambulatory setting

Drug	Induction Bolus Dose	Maintenance Infusion Rate	Maintenance Intermittent Boluses
Thiopental	5–7 mg/kg	—	—
Midazolam	Not recommended as hypnotic agent in ambulatory general anesthesia		
Etomidate	0.3 mg/kg	—	—
Propofol	2–3 mg/kg	6–10 mg/kg/h	—
Fentanyl	50–100 μg	—	25–50 μg
Alfentanil	0.5–1.5 mg	1–3 mg/h	0.2–0.5 mg
Remifentanil	1 μg/kg	0.1–0.25 μg/kg/min	—
Ketamine	0.1–0.2 mg/kg	5–10 μg/kg/min	—

From: Tesniere A, Servin F. Intravenous techniques in ambulatory anesthesia. *Anesthesiol Clin North America*. 2003; 21:273–288.

Table 9.4. Examples of dosing regimens for the various anesthetic intravenous agents during conscious sedation in the ambulatory setting

Drug	Induction Bolus Dose	Maintenance infusion Rate	Maintenance intermittent Boluses
Midazolam	1–5 mg	—	1–2 mg
Propofol	0.5–1 mg/kg	2–4 mg/kg/h	0.3–0.5 mg/kg
Fentanyl	25–50 μg	—	25–50 μg
Alfentanil	0.2–0.5 mg	0.5–2 mg/h	0.2–0.5 mg
Remifentanil	—	0.025–0.1 μg/kg/min	25 μg
Ketamine	0.1 mg/kg	2–4 μg/kg/min	—

From: Tesniere A, Servin F. Intravenous techniques in ambulatory anesthesia. *Anesthesiol Clin North America*. 2003; 21:273–288.

Inhalational agents

Inhalational anesthesia remains the most common anesthetic technique used in the ambulatory setting (see Box 9.4).

Box 9.4

The Ideal General Anesthetic Should Provide the Following:
- Smooth rapid induction
- Optimal operating conditions
- Rapid recovery
- Minimal side effects

The correct choice of an inhalational agent can help facilitate the "fast track" philosophy, enable the transfer of patients directly from the OR to the phase II recovery area, bypassing the PACU. Each of the newer short-acting inhaled anesthetics (e.g., desflurane and sevoflurane) is tolerated well by patients, achieves a rapid depth of anesthesia, has minimal side effects and metabolism, and permits rapid patient awakening. Studies have shown that propofol, sevoflurane, and desflurane facilitate rapid emergence from anesthesia, and there was no difference in recovery endpoints such as home readiness and actual time for discharge. In a study comparing the recovery profile of propofol versus desflurane and sevoflurane, it was observed in a 10-year review of the literature that PONV was significantly more common with the inhaled agents compared with propofol (6,7).

A meta-analysis of randomized controlled studies published before 1994 examined the differences in recovery time (e.g., emergence and home readiness) with desflurane and isoflurane (eight studies) and with desflurane and propofol (six studies) (8). Compared with isoflurane, desflurane was associated with a faster emergence (mean difference of 4.4 minutes). There were no differences in emergence time between desflurane and propofol (8). Immediate recovery after anesthesia with sevoflurane is faster compared with propofol and isoflurane, although this did not translate to an earlier discharge from the PACU. There was no difference in the time-to-home readiness between the different agents (9,10). These results were confirmed by a meta-analysis of randomized controlled studies (11).

Song et al. (12) assessed the recovery times and ability to fast track with desflurane, sevoflurane, or propofol. Compared with propofol total intravenous anesthesia (TIVA), maintenance of anesthesia with desflurane and sevoflurane resulted in shorter times to awakening, tracheal extubation, and orientation. A significantly larger percentage of patients who received desflurane for maintenance were considered fast-track eligible compared with sevoflurane and propofol (90% vs 75% vs 26% respectively) (12). There was no difference between the groups with respect to the times to oral intake and home readiness.

A Comment on Nitrous Oxide (N_2O)

Nitrous oxide N_2O is routinely used as a part of a balanced anesthetic because of its amnestic analgesic properties as well as its ability to reduce the requirements of inhaled or intravenous anesthetic drugs. There are several studies that have suggested that N_2O increases the incidence of PONV. The fact is that a meta-analysis of randomized controlled trials found that the emetic effect of N_2O is not significant (13).

The use of N_2O reduces the time to spontaneous breathing after equi-MAC (1.3 MAC) regimens of sevoflurane (14). A large study in women undergoing outpatient gynecologic surgery compared the incidence of PONV and the time-to-home readiness with propofol-N_2O and propofol-alone anesthetic techniques (15). The results indicate that the use of N_2O reduced the propofol requirements by 20% to 25% without increasing the incidence of adverse events or the time-to-home readiness (16). Most studies evaluating the feasibility of fast tracking after outpatient surgery have used N_2O as part of their anesthetic technique (15,17,18). There appears to be no convincing reason to avoid N_2O in the office setting.

Propofol

Most outpatient surgical facilities prefer propofol as the drug of choice for induction and maintenance of day-case anesthesia. Because of its favorable pharmacokinetic and pharmacodynamic profile, it is currently the most widely used intravenous agent for ambulatory anesthesia and sedation. It can be used solely or as part of TIVA, by intermittent boluses, or by continuous infusions (3). Propofol is easy to administer, it has a rapid onset, a short duration of action, a low incidence of PONV, and high patient acceptance. In addition, propofol is associated with a more rapid recovery of cognitive function, less postoperative sedation, less drowsiness, and less confusion. Equilibrium half-life between plasma and effect site is less than 3 minutes (19). Its context-sensitive half-life, a high plasma clearance (equal or greater than liver blood flow), associated with a large volume of distribution, results in a fast awakening even after prolonged continuous infusions when propofol is used as the sole anesthetic agent. When used at subhypnotic doses, propofol provides a titratable level of sedation, with anxiolysis and amnesia similar to that of midazolam (20). At low doses, its minimal respiratory effects allow spontaneous ventilation during the maintenance of sedation and anesthesia (3).

Because propofol falls into the chemical subclass of alcohols, patients tend to wake up in a more pleasant, at times "euphoric" state. In terms of fast-track anesthesia, because of its direct antiemetic effects (21), the incidence of PONV in the PACU is low with propofol (22) (see Table 9.5).

One study compared sevoflurane-N_2O to propofol-N_2O in fast-track office-based anesthesia (7). More than 100 patients undergoing superficial surgical procedures at an office-based surgical center were randomly assigned to one of three groups. In group I, propofol 2 mg per kg was given for induction and followed by propofol at 75 to 150 $\mu g/kg/min$ with N_2O 67% in oxygen for maintenance anesthesia. In group II, propofol 2 mg per kg was given for induction and followed by sevoflurane with N_2O 67% in oxygen for maintenance anesthesia. In group III, anesthesia was induced and maintained with sevoflurane

Table 9.5.   Clinical and adverse effects of propofol

Propofol	
Clinical Effects	Adverse Effects
• Sedation[a] • Hypnosis[a] • Anxiolysis[a] • Muscle relaxation[a] • ↓ ICP[a] • ↓ Cerebral metabolic rate[a] • Antiemetic[b]	• Respiratory depression (exacerbated by opioids)[a] • Hypotension[a] • Decreased myocardial contractility[c] • Preservative issues[d] • Potential for infection[d] • Tolerance[e] • Propofol infusion syndrome[f] • ↑ Serum triglycerides[d]

[a]Harvey MA. *Am J Crit Care*. 1996; 5:7–16.
[b]Apfel CC, et al. *Anaesthesist*. 2005; 54:201–9.
[c]Lerch C, et al. *Br Med Bull*. 1999; 55:76–95.
[d]Diprivan [package insert]. AstraZeneca Pharmaceuticals; 2004.
[e]Zapantis A, et al. *Crit Care Nurs Clin N Am*. 2005; 17:211–223.
[f]Riker RR, et al. *Pharmacotherapy*. 2005;25(5 Pt 2):8S–18S.

in combination with N_2O 67% in oxygen. Local anesthetic was used at the incision site. Comparison of the three groups showed that time to tolerating fluids, recovery room stay, and discharge times were significantly decreased when propofol was used for both induction and maintenance. The incidence of PONV and the need for rescue antiemetics were also reduced with propofol anesthesia. In addition, total costs and patient satisfaction were more favorable with propofol used for induction and maintenance of anesthesia.

Since its invention, propofol has become somewhat of a wonder drug that is an ultra short-acting sedative hypnotic, which enables the fast-track on-and-off phenomenon regarding sedation. Initially, its use was limited to those members of the anesthesia care team. Because of its ease in administration and its rapid, short-acting onset without cumulative sedative effects, propofol is being used by other medical personnel outside the recommended anesthesia care team. Who should and who should not administer propofol has become a controversial issue, given that patient safety is at stake. In 2004, the ASA issued a *Statement on Safe Use of Propofol* (23) (see Appendix 2). It recognizes that each patient may respond differently to propofol, and that each patient should receive care consistent with that required for deep sedation. The statement also addresses the need for proper training for the anesthesia provider, so that the provider can properly take care of the patient if deeper-than-intended sedation occurs (see Box 9.5).

Box 9.5

During the administration of propofol, patients should be monitored without interruption to assess level of consciousness, and to identify early signs of hypotension, bradycardia, apnea, airway obstruction, and/or oxygen desaturation. Ventilation, oxygen saturation, heart rate, and blood pressure should be monitored at regular and frequent intervals. Monitoring for the presence of

> **Box 9.5** *Continued*
> exhaled carbon dioxide should be utilized when possible, as movement of the
> chest will not dependably identify airway obstruction or apnea.

The three most common types of procedures that are performed in the office-based setting are GI, ophthalmology, and plastic surgery. Because of the historic safety profile of propofol and the cost−benefit incentives involved, many specialists are seeking to add propofol to their "sedation" protocol without the use of anesthesiology personnel. Therefore the onus is on our profession to create more specific guidelines for nonanesthesiologists as they continue to routinely use propofol in their offices.

Opioids

Opioids have been used with local anesthesia to decrease the pain associated with the injection of local anesthetics as well as the discomfort from nonincisional factors such as back pain secondary to lying on an OR table and traction on deep tissues not rendered insensitive by local anesthetic solutions. Opioids do not reliably produce sedation by themselves. When combined with other sedatives in even small amounts, opioids can cause respiratory depression. Other side effects of opioids are nausea, vomiting, and pruritus. A number of common opioids are described in the subsequent text.

Fentanyl is the most commonly used opioid during intravenous sedation. It has a fast onset (3 to 5 minutes) and its duration of action is 45 to 60 minutes (at lower doses). The typical bolus dose is 25 to 50 μg. At higher doses, cumulative effects of fentanyl are seen due to saturation of peripheral binding sites, after which the pharmacokinetics more closely resemble that of a longer-acting narcotic (e.g., morphine). At this point, fentanyl then carries a higher risk of sedation and respiratory depression.

Alfentanil is a more rapid acting analog of fentanyl. It can be given by intermittent boluses or by continuous infusion. The bolus dose is in the range of 0.25 to 0.75 mg, and the infusion dose is in the range of 0.5 to 3.0 μg/kg/min. No cumulative effects of the drug are seen when the infusion pump is discontinued.

Remifentanil is a potent short-acting opioid analgesic. It is metabolized by a nonspecific plasma and tissue esterase. This is important because metabolism is not dependent on the liver or kidney; therefore, remifentanil is an ideal drug to use in patients with kidney or liver disease. It is rapidly eliminated from the body and does not accumulate when administered by continuous infusion. The half-life is 3 to 5 minutes and is largely independent of the duration of infusion. The advantage of such a short-acting drug is the ability to provide analgesia intraoperatively without postoperative sedation or drowsiness. The bolus dose for remifentanil is in the range of 12.5 to 25 μg. The infusion dose range is 0.025 to 0.20 μg/kg/min (2). One disadvantage of remifentanil is its short duration of residual analgesia following painful procedures; therefore, local anesthesia or a nonsteroidal anti-inflammatory drug (NSAID) must be used for postoperative pain control (24).

Nonopioid Analgesics

Nonopioid analgesics prevent pain by decreasing the synthesis of prostaglandin. Prostaglandins sensitize the pain receptors to any injury (e.g., surgical incision). In addition, the nonsteroidal anti-inflammatory medications decrease the requirement for opioids, thereby decreasing the opioid side effects. Ketorolac is the commonly used parenterally active NSAID. It is associated with a decreased incidence of nausea, vomiting, and pruritus compared with fentanyl. Its standard IV dose is from 15 to 30 mg. Because

Table 9.6.   Table of nonsteroidal anti-inflammatory drugs and acetaminophen (adults)

Drug	Dose	Onset	Duration
Acetaminophen	650–1,000 mg PO q 4–6 h to max 4 g/24 h	30 min	4 h
Ibuprofen	200–400 mg q4–6 to max 3.2 g/24 h	30 min to 1 h	4–6 h
Ketorolac	Single-dose treatment: 30–60 mg IM or 15–30 mg IV	IM: 30 min IV: 10–20 min	IM/IV: 4–6 h
	Multiple-dose treatment: 15–30 mg IM or IV q4–6 hr to max 40 mg/day		
	Oral: 10 mg q4–6 h to max 40 mg/day	Oral: 30 min	Oral: 5–6 h
Indomethacin	25–50 mg/dose 2–3 times/day to max 200 mg/day	within 30 min	4–6 h
Celecoxib	100–400 mg twice per day	45 min	6–8 h

From: Redmond M, Florence B, Class PS. Effective analgesic modalities for ambulatory patients. *Anesthesiol Clin North Am.* 2003; 21:329–346.

prostaglandins are involved in the maintenance of blood flow to the kidney, maintenance of the lining of the stomach, and the normal function of platelets involved in the clotting process, *NSAIDs should be used with caution in patients with kidney problems, GI problems, and bleeding disorders.* Celecoxib is another alternative to the traditional NSAIDs, with less effect on the platelet function and GI lining. Acetaminophen, an inhibitor of prostaglandin synthesis, is another drug class important in multimodal pain therapy and pre-emptive surgical analgesia (see Table 9.6).

α_2 Agonists

α_2 Agonists, such as clonidine and dexmedetomidine (DEX), are a unique class of drugs that were originally used as nasal decongestants and were used in the treatment of hypertension. A preservative-free form was synthesized in the early 1990s. When injected intravenously or epidurally, it was found to prolong the effects of local anesthetics and narcotics. α_2 Agonists act in the CNS by decreasing sympathetic nervous system outflow and also have profound sedative, anxiolytic, and analgesic effects. Studies of this unique class of non-narcotic agents show that their use decreases the requirement of anesthetic (inhalation) and other sedatives (intravenous or epidural). In addition to these benefits, this class of drug maintains cardiovascular and respiratory stability, making it a very attractive drug to use in the office-based setting.

The newest drug in this class is DEX, and it appears to be an excellent adjuvant to use in cases that require intravenous sedation. Similar to all other α_2 agonists, DEX decreases the requirement of other sedatives in order to minimize potential side effects, maintains spontaneous ventilation, and maintains cardiovascular stability. DEX is generally initiated with a loading dose of 1 μg per kg over 10 minutes, which is followed by an infusion dose of 0.2 to 0.7 μg/kg/hr. The distribution half-life is 9 minutes and the elimination half-life is approximately 2 hours. DEX pharmacokinetics was not significantly different in patients with renal impairment compared with healthy subjects; however, clearance values for patients with hepatic failure were lower than in healthy subjects. DEX is generally well tolerated, and the most common treatment-related adverse events reported include hypotension, nausea, bradycardia, and dry mouth (25).

Because of its anxiolytic, sedative, analgesic, sympatholytic, and amnestic properties, DEX has significant clinical utility. It appears to be particularly safe with respect to respiratory function. Ebert et al. showed that the respiratory system remains relatively uncompromised during DEX infusions, even at high doses (26). Continuous infusion maintains unique sedation (patients appear to be asleep, but are readily roused), analgesic sparing effect, and minimal depression of respiratory drive. Experiments have shown anxiolytic effects in humans using intramuscular doses of 2.4 μg per kg and potentiation of the anxiolytic effect of midazolam in rats (27). Finally, it provided some immediate (not retrograde) memory impairment (28). Ebert et al. also demonstrated that DEX at low-dose infusions (0.2–0.8 μg/kg/min) lowered the mean arterial pressure by 13% (26). One plausible explanation is that plasma levels of norepinephrine were decreased by 60% to 85%, thereby blunting the sympathetic response during the perioperative period. In addition, intramuscular or intravenous administration of DEX induced bradycardia and caused a decrease in cardiac output in a dose-dependent manner. The drug seemed to produce its cardiac depressant effects through activation of the brain α_2 adrenoceptors, resulting in inhibition of the vasomotor center and the consequent decrease in the central sympathetic drive reaching the heart and the blood vessels through the spinal cord. Furthermore, the ability of DEX to induce diuresis and to enhance sodium excretion may contribute to its hypotensive action (25). The hemodynamic effects of DEX related to its α_2 agonist properties are of potential clinical benefit. By decreasing HR, DEX contributes to an increase in coronary blood supply to the left ventricle through prolongation of diastole. The reduction in HR would be associated with decreased myocardial oxygen consumption (29). In addition, by decreasing BP, DEX may reduce procedure-related blood loss.

Recently, we performed a retrospective study evaluating 170 patients who received intravenous sedation with DEX (30). DEX appears to be a safe and effective anesthetic for patients undergoing aesthetic facial surgery. The key issue that led to our use of DEX is the added safety to the patients. The cardiorespiratory effects of DEX combine intravenous sedation while allowing the patient to breathe room air spontaneously without the use of supplemental oxygen. This effect avoids the issue of combustion seen with the combination of oxygen and electrocautery/laser commonly used during facial surgery.

DEX has much promise in the outpatients receiving MAC anesthesia, because it provides safety for patients intraoperatively and also decreases the amount of pain medications used postoperatively. It is a drug that fits perfectly with the "fast track" philosophy. As of 2007, there are multi-institutional phase III U.S. Food and Drug Administration (FDA) studies scheduled to evaluate the use of DEX in cases performed under MAC anesthesia. On the basis of the results of the forthcoming studies, we hope to provide evidence to support the routine use of DEX in the outpatient setting.

DRUG COMBINATIONS

The most commonly used drugs for office-based anesthesia are outlined individually in the preceding text. In the office-based OR setting, the common practice is to use combinations of drugs to facilitate fast-track anesthesia and MAC (see Box 9.6). We describe a few examples in the subsequent text.

Box 9.6

Examples:

1. Dexmedetomidine technique
2. Remifentanil/propofol technique
3. Ketamine/midazolam technique

Because of the consistent safety and efficacy we have seen with the addition of DEX to TIVA, the cardiorespiratory and MAC sparing benefits make this technique an ideal template for "challenging patients" in various types of surgical scenarios. We present the drug regimen and technique using the aesthetic facial surgical patient as an example (30).

- Midazolam 2 to 4 mg IV in the holding area; an additional 2 to 4 mg IV can be given in the OR.
- All IV anesthetics and analgesics are diluted to a base of "10": 10 μg/mL (DEX, fentanyl) or 10 mg per mL (propofol, ketamine).
- Once in the OR, while the ASA standard monitors are being placed, loading doses of DEX (1 μg/kg) and ketamine (0.25−0.75 mg/kg) over 10 to 15 minutes are started.
- A urinary catheter is placed at the completion of the loading dose; the lack of movement or verbal response during urinary catheter placement is a good indication that an adequate level of sedation had been achieved for the forthcoming facial injection of local anesthetic.
- A DEX infusion is continued at 0.2 to 0.7 μg/kg/hr and a ketamine infusion is continued at 10 to 50 μg/kg/min.
- A propofol infusion of 10 to 30 μg/kg/min is started during the sterile preparation and drape and titrated based on the patient's response to the injection of local anesthetic into the desired surgical area.
- If the patient is unable to tolerate the local anesthetic injection, 1 to 2 mL of DEX (10 μg/mL) and 1 to 2 mL of ketamine (10 mg/mL) are bolused.
- In refractory patients, 1 to 2 mL of fentanyl (10 μg/mL) can be given and titrated to the patient's respiratory rate.
- Midazolam 1 to 2 mg IV every 1 to 2 hours can be given to maintain amnesia.
- The patient typically undergoes this anesthetic without supplemental oxygen. In the event of desaturation, the surgeon is asked to hold the electrocautery, and to perform a jaw-thrust maneuver. If the oxygen desaturation remains, supplemental oxygen is then administered by the anesthesia personnel through a face mask.
- At the conclusion of the case, all infusions are stopped when the surgical dressings are being placed. The patient is usually alert within 5 to 10 minutes and is able to move to the transport bed.

Another example is the combination of remifentanil and propofol, which has been shown to decrease mean OR time and OR plus PACU charges when compared with a conventional balanced anesthetic (24). Patients received a mixture starting at 50 μg/mL of remifentanil and 10 mg/mL of propofol that resulted in a final syringe admixture of a 20 mL solution containing 25 μg per mL of remifentanil and 5 mg per mL of propofol. The diluent was 5% dextrose and water because it is compatible with both drugs. Inductions used a slow infusion on 1.0 to 1.5 mg per kg of propofol from the mixture. The maintenance infusion was 25 to 75 μg/kg/min of propofol using the mixture. Nitrous oxide N_2O and oxygen were used in a 50/50 concentration for maintenance. Rocuronium was used if needed for intubation. Postoperative pain was controlled with a field block or ketorolac 30 to 60 mg before the end of anesthesia. Total surgery time was 27 minutes compared with 34 minutes in the conventional group, PACU time was less, and a few patients were even able to bypass the PACU entirely. In addition, OR drug charges, actual OR charges, and actual PACU charges were also decreased.

Another technique for day surgery used low-dose ketamine with clonidine and midazolam (31). Before induction of anesthesia with propofol 2 mg per kg, patients were given atropine 0.01 mg per kg, midazolam 0.03 to 0.05 mg per kg, and ketamine 0.4 mg per kg. All patients received N_2O 65% in oxygen. Vecuronium was used for muscle relaxation. Following intubation, patients were given clonidine 150 μg IV. If the depth of anesthesia was inadequate, patients were given ketamine 0.4 to 0.6 mg per kg or bolus injections of propofol 0.5 mg per kg. Ketorolac 30 mg and dexamethasone 8 mg were administered 30 minutes before wound closure. Advantages of this combination are the absence of respiratory depression and PONV, rapid awakening, rapid return of HR and BP to preoperative values, and good postoperative pain control without the use of opioids.

Propofol in combination with N_2O has been shown to decrease the anesthetic requirement for office-based surgery (18). In a group of 69 patients undergoing superficial surgical procedures lasting 15 to 45 minutes, a standard propofol induction was performed (1.5 mg/kg) followed by maintenance with propofol (100 μg/kg/min) in combination with either air of N_2O in 65% oxygen. The propofol rate was then adjusted to provide an appropriate depth of anesthesia. For all patients, local anesthetic was used at the surgical site, and no prophylactic antiemetics were given. For both groups, recovery time and the incidence of PONV were similar. In the N_2O group, the amount of propofol maintenance was decreased by 19%. All of the patients in the N_2O-propofol group were "very satisfied" with their anesthetic experience.

For MAC cases, midazolam 1 to 3 mg IV followed by a propofol infusion in the range of 10 to 100 μg/kg/min provides excellent anxiolysis, amnesia, and sedation. Recovery times are not significantly increased when compared with using propofol alone (32). For analgesia during MAC, fentanyl 25 to 50 μg IV or Alfentanil 250 to 500 μg IV may be administered 3 minutes before the injection of local anesthetic. Small boluses of fentanyl 25 μg IV or Alfentanil 250 μg IV may be given for pain that does not respond to supplemental local anesthetic. For elderly patients, doses should be decreased with midazolam dosed 0.5 to 1.0 mg IV, fentanyl 12.5 μg IV, and Alfentanil 125 μg IV (2).

An alternative for MAC cases involves premedicating with midazolam 2 mg IV, followed with an infusion of propofol 25 to 50 μg per kg in combination with remifentanil 12.5 to 25 μg bolus injections, or an infusion of 0.025 to 0.15 μg/kg/min. The potential of this combination is to utilize the sedative and antiemetic effects of propofol with the analgesic effects of remifentanil in order to decrease requirements for sedation, analgesia, and postoperative side effects (2).

MANAGEMENT OF POSTOPERATIVE NAUSEA AND VOMITING

Unplanned hospital admission in outpatient surgery results primarily from uncontrolled pain, nausea, and vomiting. Studies have clearly shown that patient satisfaction depends on avoidance of PONV in addition to a good surgical outcome. If untreated, 30% of all patients who undergo surgery will experience PONV. This is a very high number considering the number of patients undergoing outpatient procedures. Patients at the highest risk are shown in Box 9.7.

Box 9.7

Females
Middle-aged patients
Nonsmokers
Patients with history of motion sickness
Patients with history of PONV
The use of postoperative opioids

The New England Journal of Medicine published an article in 2004 looking at interventions that are the safest, most economic, and most efficient means of controlling PONV (33). A total of 5,199 patients were evaluated comparing general anesthesia with inhalation agents versus intravenous anesthesia. In terms of TIVA, the use of propofol, room air, and the ultrashort-acting narcotic remifentanil decreased the incidence of PONV. An injection of a small dose of dexamethasone was recommended to be the first-line treatment, and drugs in the serotonin antagonist class of medications such as ondansetron, granisetron, and dolansetron should be used as rescue treatment.

DRUG SAFETY IN OFFICE-BASED ANESTHESIA

Patient safety in the office-based setting is of utmost importance because safety systems taken for granted in hospital-based operating facilities are not necessarily regulated in the office. The anesthesiologist may need to exercise greater vigilance to insure that medication errors do not occur. The Closed Claims Study looked at 14 of 5,480 claims from the office-based setting. The reason for the small number of claims is due to the 3- to 5-year delay for malpractice claims to be resolved and appear in the Closed Claims database (34), the data evaluated was from 2002, the increase in office-based practice has been relatively recent (an increase in the number of cases from 5 to 10 million from 1995–2005), and a uniform method of reporting anesthesia "mishaps" has yet to be established. What can be said about the 14 claims is summarized in Box 9.8.

Box 9.8

Most of the cases involved the following:
Middle-aged women
    ASA 1–2 patients
    Elective surgeries
    General anesthesia or MAC (34).
The most common procedure in the office-based setting was plastic surgery (64%) followed by dental procedures (21%) (34).

When the *office-based anesthesia claims* were compared with the claims from the ambulatory surgical setting, the office-based claims had a *higher proportion of deaths (64%) versus ambulatory surgery claims (21%). The most common damaging event was the respiratory system (50%)* including bronchospasm, airway obstruction, inadequate oxygenation and/or ventilation, and esophageal intubation. *Drug-related damaging events* included the following:

- Administration of the wrong drug
- Administration of the incorrect dosage of the drug
- Malignant hyperthermia (34)

Owing to these issues, the ASA has issued standards on the proper labeling of drugs used in the operative setting. These are outlined in the appendixes at the end of the book, and are also available on the ASA website (see Appendix 3).

CONCLUSION

Patient satisfaction is high on the list of priorities, and this is especially true in the office-based OR setting. Satisfaction is dependent on a good surgical outcome in addition to adequate analgesia, and avoidance of PONV. What has been found in many questionnaires sent to patients postoperatively is that patient satisfaction depends on the number of these minor "setbacks," and as the number increases, satisfaction decreases (35). In the current era of medicine, patient safety, cost efficiency along with high-quality "patient friendly" service, and patient satisfaction are essential components of a successful office-based surgical practice. The marketplace demands it, and patients are increasingly discerning about the quality and level of care that they choose (see Box 9.9).

Box 9.9

The office:

Affordable, Safe, Patient-Centered

+

The patient:

Adequate Pain Control, Avoidance of PONV, Attention to Detail, Privacy

=

PATIENT SATISFACTION

So which drugs make the "best pharmacologic cocktail?" This type of anesthesia is not as easy, simple, and straightforward as one might think. It is a balance between creativity, safety, and patient satisfaction. There is no one cookbook formula for the anesthetic plan because it is derived on an individual basis. If several anesthesiologists are asked how they would provide anesthesia for a specific patient, the majority would agree on the key issues and drugs required; however, one anesthesiologist questioned might have his or her own specific preferences based on experience, knowledge, and comfort level. There are several routes to achieve the same goal in each patient. The first step is the discussion between the patient and anesthesiologist (anesthesia personnel). With this in mind, the best plan is the one that will ensure the safest, most pleasant, and comfortable experience.

REFERENCES

1. Crews J. Multimodal pain management strategies for office-based and ambulatory procedures. *JAMA*. 2002;288(5):629–632.
2. Sa Rego MM, Watcha MF, White PF. The changing role of monitored anesthesia care in the ambulatory setting. *Anesth Anal*. 1997;85:1020–1036.
3. Tesniere A, Servin F. Intravenous techniques in ambulatory anesthesia. *Anesthesiol Clin North America*. 2003;21:273–288.
4. Suzuki M, Tsueda K, Lansing PS, et al. Midazolam attenuates ketamine-induced abnormal perception and thought process but not mood changes. *Can J Anesthesiol*. 2000;47(9):866–874.
5. Cillo JE. Propofol anesthesia for outpatient oral and maxillofacial surgery. *Oral Surg Oral Med Oral Pathol Oral Radiol Endod*. 1999;87:530–538.

6. Gupta A. Comparison of recovery profile after ambulatory anesthesia with propofol, isoflurane, sevoflurane, and desflurane: A systematic review. *Anesth Analg*. 2004;98(3):632–641.
7. Tang J. Recovery profile, costs, and patient satisfaction with propofol and sevoflurane for fast-track office-based anesthesia. *Anesthesiology*. 1999;91(1): 253–261.
8. Dexter F, Tinker JH. Comparison between desflurane and isoflurane or propofol on time to following commands and time to discharge. A Meta-Analysis. *Anesthesiology*. 1995;83:77–82.
9. Fredman B, Nathanson MH, Smith I, et al. Sevoflurane for outpatient anesthesia: A comparison with propofol. *Anesth Analg*. 1995;81:823–828.
10. Raeder J, et al. Recovery characteristics of sevoflurane- or propofol-based anaesthesia for day-care surgery. *Acta Anaesthesiol Scand*. 1997;41:988–994.
11. Robinson BJ, et al. A review of recovery from sevoflurane anaesthesia: Comparison with isoflurane and propofol including meta-analysis. *Acta Anaesthesiol Scand*. 1999;43:185–190.
12. Song D, Joshi GP, White PF, et al. Fast-track eligibility after ambulatory anesthesia: A comparison of desflurane, sevoflurane, and propofol. *Anesth Analg*. 1998;86:267–273.
13. Tramer M, et al. Omitting nitrous oxide in general anaesthesia: Meta-analysis of intraoperative awareness and postoperative emesis in randomized controlled trials. *Br J Anaesth*. 1996;76:186–193.
14. Einarsson S, et al. Decreased respiratory depression during emergence from anesthesia with sevoflurane/N_2O than with sevoflurane alone. *Can J Anaesth*. 1999;46:335–341.
15. Arellano RJ, et al. Omission of nitrous oxide from a propofol-based anesthetic does not affect the recovery of women undergoing outpatient gynecological surgery. *Anesthesiology*. 2000;93:332–339.
16. Joshi GP. Recent developments in regional anesthesia for ambulatory surgery. *Curr Opin Anaesthesiol*. 1999;12:643–647.
17. Johnson GW, St John Gray H. Nitrous oxide inhalation as an adjunct to intravenous induction of general anesthesia with propofol for day surgery. *Eur J Anaesthesiol*. 1997;14:295–299.
18. Tang J, et al. Use of propofol for office-based anesthesia: Effect of nitrous oxide on recovery profile. *J Clin Anesth*. 1999;11:226–230.
19. Schnider TW, et al. The influence of age on propofol pharmacodynamics. *Anesthesiology*. 1999;90:1502–1516.
20. Veselis RA, et al. The comparative amnestic effects of midazolam, propofol, thiopental and fentanyl at equisedative concentrations. *Anesthesiology*. 1997;87:749–764.
21. Borgeat A. Subhyptonic doses of propofol possess direct antiemetic properties. *Anesth Analg*. 1992;74:539–541.
22. Joo HS, Perks WJ. Sevoflurane versus propofol for anesthetic induction: A meta-analysis. *Anesth Analg*. 2000;91:213–219.
23. American Society of Anesthesiologists. ASA statement of safe use of propofol. Approved by the ASA House of Delegates; Available at: http://www.asahq.org/publicationsAndServices/standards/37.pdf. 2004.
24. Brady W. Use of remifentanil and propofol combination in outpatients to facilitate rapid discharge home. *AANA J*. 2005;73(3):207–210.
25. El-Tahir kel-D. Dexmedetomidine: A sedative-analgesic drug for the 21st century. *Middle East J Anesthesiol*. 2002;16(6):577–585.
26. Ebert T, Hall JE, Barney JA, et al. The effects of increasing plasma concentrations of dexmedetomidine in humans. *Anesthesiology*. 2000;93:382–394.
27. Salonen M, et al. Dexmedetomidine synergism with midazolam in the elevated plus-maze test in rats. *Psychopharmacology*. 1992;108:229–243.
28. Hall JE, et al. Sedative, amnestic, and analgesic properties of small-dose dexmedetomidine infusions. *Anesth Analg*. 2000;90:699–705.

29. Mantz J, et al. Phase III study on dexmedetomidine used for postoperative sedation of patients requiring mechanical ventilation for less than 24 hours: The French experience. *Middle East J Anesthesiol.* 2002;16(6):597–606.

30. Taghinia AH, et al. Dexmedetomidine in facial aesthetic surgery: Improving anesthetic safety and efficacy. *Plast Reconstr Surg.* In press.

31. Dalsasso M. Low-dose ketamine with clonidine and midazolam for adult day care surgery. *Eur J Anaesthesiol.* 2005;22:67–79.

32. Taylor E. Midazolam in combination with propofol for sedation during local anesthesia. *J Clin Anesth.* 1992;4:213–216.

33. Apfel C. A factorial trial of six interventions for the prevention of postoperative nausea and vomiting. *N Engl J Med.* 2004;350(24):2441–2451.

34. Lee LA. The closed claims project. Has it influenced anesthetic practice and outcome? *Anesthesiol Clin North America.* 2002;20(3):485–501.

35. Coyle T, Helfrick JF, Gonzalez ML, et al. Ambulatory anesthesia: Factors that influence patient satisfaction or dissatisfaction with deep sedation or general anesthesia. *J Maxillofac Surg.* 2005;63:163–172.

Monitors

Alexander C. Gerhart

Twenty-first century anesthesia providers are increasingly being asked to provide anesthesia care in office-based environments. Under ideal circumstances, the cases involve healthy American Society of Anesthesiologists (ASA) class 1 patients undergoing minor surgical procedures with low potential for complication. Although risk can be minimized through proper patient selection, adequate training, and vigilance, it cannot be eliminated. The use of proper patient monitors coupled with the experience of a trained anesthesia provider can detect potential adverse events, prevent complications, and minimize morbidity. The ASA mandates that all anesthetics, whether general, regional, or monitored anesthesia care (MAC) be provided under *The Standards for Anesthetic Monitoring* (http://www.asahq.org/publicationsAndServices/standards/02.pdf) (see Appendix 4). Standard I states that adequately trained personnel provide the anesthetic. Standard II states that for all anesthetics, the patient's oxygenation, circulation, ventilation, and temperature shall be continually monitored (see Box 10.1). The next few pages will describe the current monitoring devices available, as well as look toward the future of monitoring techniques as they pertain to office-based anesthesia.

Box 10.1 • ASA-Mandated Monitoring

Oxygenation
Circulation
Ventilation
Temperature

OXYGENATION

1. During every administration of general anesthesia using an anesthesia machine, the concentration of oxygen in the breathing system shall be measured by an oxygen analyzer with a low oxygen concentration limit alarm in use (see Box 10.2).

Box 10.2

Concentration of inspired oxygen is measured with oxygen analyzer.
Oxygenation is measured by pulse oximetry.

---

2. During all anesthetics, a quantitative method of assessing oxygenation such as pulse oximetry shall be employed (see Figure 10.1).

There are several types of oxygen analyzers in commercial use on modern anesthesia machines. The most common is the galvanic cell, which is composed of a lead anode and a gold cathode bathed in potassium chloride. The lead anode is consumed by hydroxyl ions formed at the gold cathode forming lead oxide and producing a current. This current can be measured and the inspired oxygen content calculated based on the current generated. The lead anode of galvanic (fuel) cells is constantly being degraded, and fuel cell life can be prolonged by exposing them to room air when not in use. Other less common techniques for measuring inspired oxygen content include paramagnetic analysis and polarographic electrodes.

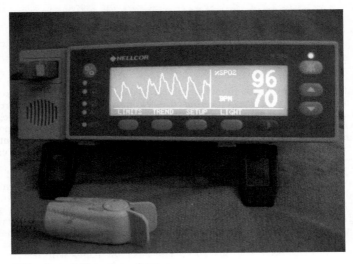

Figure 10.1.　A portable pulse oximeter.

The use of pulse oximetry is mandatory for all patients undergoing an anesthetic. There are no contraindications to its use. Pulse oximetry is based on a sensor containing either two or three light sources (light emitting diodes), and one light detector (photodiode). Hemoglobin saturation is calculated based on the knowledge that oxyhemoglobin (960 nm) and deoxyhemoglobin (660 nm) absorb light at different wavelengths. The ratio of light absorbed at each wavelength provides the measure of hemoglobin saturation. Many factors may confound pulse oximeter readings (see Box 10.3). Carboxyhemoglobin, which occurs in the setting of carbon monoxide (CO) poisoning, absorbs light at the same wavelength as oxyhemoglobin and therefore yields artificially elevated readings. Methemoglobinemia absorbs light at both 660 and 990 nm, and yields a pulse oximeter reading of 85%. Other common causes of spurious pulse oximeter readings include ambient light interference, decreased perfusion, decreased cardiac output, increased systemic vascular resistance, peripheral vascular disease, and motion artifact. Patients will often present for office-based anesthetics with nail polish or artificial nails, which may affect the quality of pulse oximetry tracings. Nail polish is easily removed with acetone or the oximeter may be placed on a toe, or an ear. Another option would be to use a disposable oximeter sensor that can be placed on the nose or forehead.

Box 10.3

Common Causes of Abnormal Pulse Oximetry Values
Carboxyhemoglobin
Methemoglobin
Ambient light interference
Decreased perfusion (increased systemic vascular resistance, decreased CO, peripheral vascular disease)
Motion artifact
Artificial fingernail applications
Nail polish

The use of pulse oximetry and oxygen analyzers cannot be disputed, but they must be considered the starting point for the monitoring of oxygenation. The anesthesia provider must also note subjective cues of inadequate oxygenation in the awake patient, including change in mentation and dyspnea (see Box 10.4). Additionally, adequate lighting and exposure of the patient are required to allow inspection and assessment of color and skin tone. In the discussion on monitoring oxygenation, it is worthwhile to mention the need to ensure the adequacy of the primary oxygen supply and the presence of a reserve oxygen supply. The importance of ensuring an adequate oxygen supply cannot be overstated. There have been several reported fatalities occurring during the administration of anesthesia in office-based settings in which patients died of respiratory failure in locations without supplemental oxygen available.

Box 10.4

Subjective Assessment of Oxygenation
Change in mentation
Complaints of dyspnea
Pallor
Cyanosis

VENTILATION

1. Every patient receiving general anesthesia shall have the adequacy of ventilation continually evaluated (see Box 10.5).

Box 10.5

Assessment of Adequate Ventilation
End-tidal CO_2 monitor
Capnography tracing
Disconnect alarm for circuit
Physical examination and observation of chest wall movement
Presence of condensation on a face mask or inside an endotracheal tube
Auscultation of breath sounds (precordial stethoscope)

---

2. When a tracheal tube or laryngeal mask airway is inserted, correct position must be verified by the presence of end-tidal CO_2. The continued presence of end-tidal CO_2 will be quantitatively measured from the time of endotracheal tube/laryngeal mask airway insertion, until its removal, or transfer of the patient to a postoperative location.
3. When ventilation is controlled by a mechanical ventilator, there shall be in continuous use a device capable of detecting disconnection of components of the breathing system.
4. During regional anesthesia and MAC, the adequacy of ventilation shall be evaluated, at least, by continual observation of qualitative clinical signs.

The simplest techniques for monitoring ventilation include inspection, auscultation, and palpation. For regional anesthesia or MAC, monitoring ventilation may simply include listening to the respiratory pattern and rate and observation of chest excursion. The addition of a capnography sampling line to a nasal cannula or face mask provides qualitative indications of respiratory rate and effectiveness in wave form. A precordial stethoscope may also be employed although awake patients may complain of its weight, and many anesthesia providers object to being physically tethered to a patient.

For a patient undergoing a general anesthetic, it is imperative that end-tidal CO_2 is continuously monitored and it is strongly encouraged that the

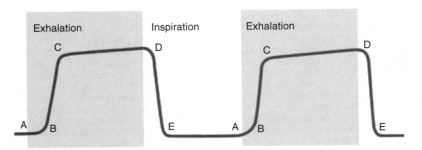

Figure 10.2. A normal capnogram.
A–B: Exhalation of CO_2 free gas contained in dead space at the beginning of exhalation.
B–C: Respiratory upstroke, representing the emptying of connecting airways and the beginning of emptying of alveoli.
C–D: Expiratory (or alveolar) plateau, representing emptying of alveoli—due to uneven emptying of alveoli, the slope continues to rise gradually during the expiratory pause.
D: End-tidal CO_2 level—the best approximation of alveolar CO_2 level.
D–E: Inspiratory downstroke, as the patient begins to inhale fresh gas.
E–A: Inspiratory pause, where CO_2 remains at 0.

anesthesia provider has access to capnography tracings. Capnography tracings and end-tidal CO_2 monitoring provide clues to many pertinent clinical conditions (see Figures 10.2 and 10.3 and Box 10.6). Esophageal intubation, circuit disconnect, failure of inspiratory or expiratory vales, exhaustion of CO_2 absorbent, obstruction of the endotracheal tube, obstructive pulmonary disease, restrictive pulmonary disease, spontaneous diaphragm movement, pulmonary embolism, and malignant hyperthermia may all result in changes in the capnograph tracing. For patients undergoing procedures on the face, where oxygen cannula or mask may be contraindicated, transcutaneous CO_2 monitors are available.

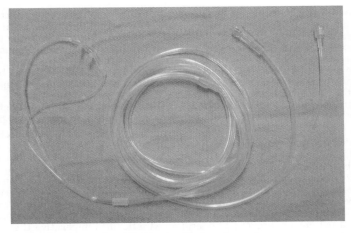

Figure 10.3. Nasal cannula with CO_2 monitoring channel.

Box 10.6

Diagnostic Clues Provided by Capnography
Restrictive lung disease
Obstructive lung disease
Esophageal intubation
Circuit disconnect
Failure of inspiratory or expiratory valves
Malignant hyperthermia
Myocardial infarction
Pulmonary embolism

Many monitors of ventilation may be part of a commercially manufactured anesthesia machine. In the office-based setting, it is important that the anesthesia provider is familiar with the function of the machine available, and is able to verify maintenance is properly performed in a timely manner. In the office-based setting, the anesthetist must ensure that anesthesia equipment and emergency equipment are maintained (see Box 10.7 and Figure 10.4). In the current medicolegal environment in which we practice, keeping a written maintenance log that details all maintenance performed and allows the provider to show compliance with manufacturers-suggested maintenance schedule is essential. Machine checkout is required before each

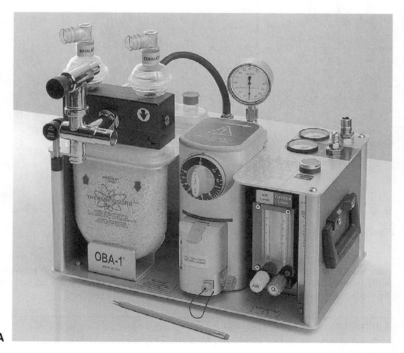

A

Figure 10.4. A: Portable anesthesia machine. B: Traditional anesthesia machine. C: Wheeled lockable storage cart to ensure all needed supplies are close at hand and easily located in an emergency.

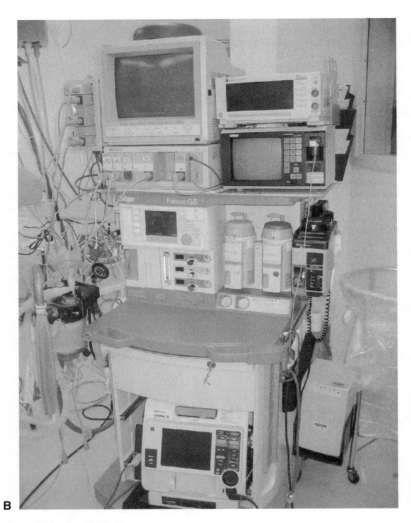

B

Figure 10.4.   (continued)

case, and a backup means of providing positive pressure ventilation must be readily available. Additionally, backup electrical power, either in the form of generator or battery, should be available (see Appendix 5).

Box 10.7

The ASA provides an excellent tool for evaluating the suitability of anesthesia machines for use.
http://www.asahq.org/publicationsAndServices/machineobsolescense.pdf

---

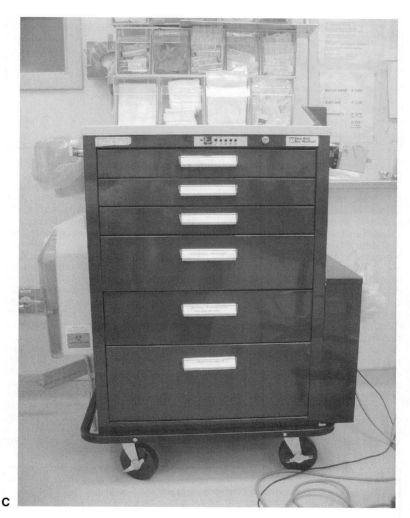

C

Figure 10.4. (continued)

CIRCULATION

1. Every patient receiving anesthesia shall have the electrocardiogram continuously displayed from the beginning of anesthesia until leaving the anesthetizing location.
2. Every patient receiving anesthesia shall have arterial blood pressure and heart rate determined and evaluated at least every 5 minutes.
3. Every patient receiving general anesthesia shall have, in addition to the the details mentioned earlier, circulatory function continually monitored by at least one of the following: palpation of pulse, auscultation of heart sounds, monitoring a tracing of intra-arterial pressure, ultrasound peripheral pulse monitoring, or pulse plethysmography or oximetry (see Box 10.8).

Box 10.8

Evaluation of Circulation
Electrocardiography
Blood pressure
Physical examination
  Pulse characteristics
  Skin tone and color
  Capillary refill
  Heart tones (gallop, murmur)
Response to fluid challenge

Continuous electrocardiography allows monitoring of pacemaker function, ischemia, and arrhythmia detection, and may provide clues to the diagnosis of electrolyte abnormalities (see Box 10.9). Proper lead placement is essential for optimal interpretation. Most commonly, three or five electrodes are used. Three electrodes, providing leads I, II, and III, and five electrodes adding the ability to monitor a precordial lead. In machines capable of monitoring two leads simultaneously, lead II, which most closely follows the axis of myocardial depolarization is most often monitored for the detection of arrhythmia, whereas V_5 is most often monitored in order to detect ischemia. Lead V_5 is selected for its location over the left ventricle; however, leads may be placed at different locations in patients with known or suspected coronary artery disease in other distributions. Along with the ability to continuously monitor the electrocardiogram, the office-based provider must be able to recognize and respond to arrhythmia. At a minimum, this requires current advanced cardiac life support (ACLS) certification, an adequate pharmacy, and a working defibrillator. In 2005, several changes were made to the ACLS algorithms. Although beyond the scope of this discussion of monitoring devices, text references from *Circulation*, as well as the website for the American Heart Association which provides free full text versions online, may be found in the references at the end of this chapter (see Appendix 6). In the office setting, trained help may be unavailable, and the anesthetist may find himself or herself not only directing, but also performing resuscitation efforts. Automated external defibrillators are simple to use and may be found in many locations, or the suite may be equipped with a traditional defibrillator. In either case, the anesthetist must be well versed in the use of the available equipment and must be able to direct others in their use (see Figure 10.5).

Box 10.9

Diagnostic Clues Provided by Electrocardiogram
Electrolyte abnormalities
Ischemia
  Inferior II, III, aVF (right coronary artery)
  Lateral I, aVL, V_5, V_6 (Left circumflex)
  Anterior V_1, V_2 (left anterior descending [LAD] septal branch)
  Anterior V_3-V_6 (LAD diagonal branch)
Arrhythmia
Pacemaker function

Monitoring the electrocardiogram provides information regarding the electrical activity of the heart, but does not ensure adequate circulation. In the most profound case, pulseless electrical activity, the electrocardiogram may be normal, but the patient is without pulse and circulation. The simplest measures of circulatory function are inspection and palpation. Strength and character of a pulse provide rapid assessment of circulation. Brief

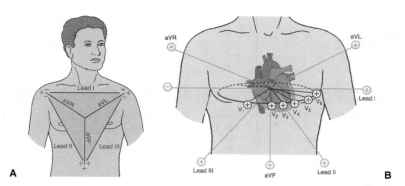

Figure 10.5. A: Electrocardiographic lead placement. B: Electrocardiographic lead vectors. In aVR, aVL, aVF, a stands for augmented, V for voltage, R for right arm, L for left arm, and F for foot.

examination of capillary refill, color, and temperature of extremities will also aid in determining a patient's circulatory status. Beyond physical examination, the simplest and most important measure of circulatory status is blood pressure measurement. The simplest method of measuring blood pressure involves placing a cuff on an extremity, inflating to a pressure greater than systolic pressure to occlude arterial flow, and palpating a distal pulse while slowly deflating the cuff. The pressure at which the pulse returns is the systolic pressure. A Doppler probe may be substituted for palpation in patients with large amounts of subcutaneous tissue, marked vasoconstriction, or weak pulse. Using a stethoscope to auscultate Korotkoff sounds, which result from turbulent flow within a vessel under a blood pressure cuff, allows determination of both systolic and diastolic pressure. In addition to these manual techniques, many devices have been developed to automatically monitor blood pressure. The most commonly used method involves detection of oscillations in blood vessels under an automatically inflated blood pressure cuff. The intensity of oscillations caused by pulsatile flow in the arterial tree changes with inflation of the cuff. Intensity is lowest when the cuff is inflated beyond systolic blood pressure, and is greatest at the mean arterial pressure. The data collected from the cuff is processed and the automated blood pressure monitor provides calculated systolic and diastolic pressures from a measured mean arterial pressure. Oscillometric techniques often fail when the pulse is irregular or systolic pressure is very low because of irregularity or decreased amplitude of oscillation within a vessel. In any cuff-based technique, selection and placement of an appropriately sized cuff is essential. The cuff width should be 120% to 150% of the diameter of the extremity on which it is placed. Placement must take into account location of intravenous lines, fistulae, lymphatic defect, and location of peripheral nerves in an effort to minimize cuff-related injury. It is also important to recognize the effect of gravity on blood pressure measurement and consider possible pathologic conditions such as coarctation of the aorta or peripheral vascular disease that may result is inaccurate blood pressure measurements.

There are several techniques for continuous blood pressure measurement (see Box 10.10). Intra-arterial monitoring is the gold standard and allows for beat-to-beat measurement of the blood pressure. Although accurate and reliable, intra-arterial catheters may be poorly tolerated and cumbersome in the office environment (see Box 10.11). Other options, although limited by patient movement, arrhythmia, and peripheral vascular disease, include tonometry and finger cuff measurement. These devices, even with their limitations, may be ideal for the office-based procedure, where the patient is likely free of arrhythmia and peripheral vascular disease. Especially when measured values can be confirmed with traditional blood pressure measurement, these alternative technologies allow for noninvasive continuous blood pressure monitoring (see Figure 10.6).

Box 10.10

Noninvasive Oscillometric Techniques for Blood Pressure Measurement
Rely upon algorithms to calculate systolic and diastolic blood pressure from measured mean arterial pressure
Are prone to failure under the following circumstances:
Too large or too small a cuff
Ideal cuff width is 120%–150% of the diameter of the limb to which the cuff is applied
Morbid obesity
Irregular heart beat (atrial fibrillation)

Box 10.11

Advantages of Invasive Blood Pressure Monitoring
Continuous measurement of "real time" pressures (allowing safe titration of vasoactive agents)
Easy access for laboratory samples (repeated arterial blood gas analysis, serial hematocrit)

Disadvantages of Invasive Blood Pressure Monitoring
May be poorly tolerated by awake unsedated patients
Potential for complication
    Hematoma
    Bleeding
    Infection
    Thrombosis
    Air embolism
    Skin or soft tissue damage at either catheter or transducer site
    Nerve injury
    Loss of distal perfusion

TEMPERATURE

Every patient receiving anesthesia shall have temperature monitored when clinically significant changes in body temperature are intended, anticipated, or expected (see Box 10.12).

Box 10.12

Hypothermia
Most often due to heat loss to the environment
Elderly patients may have a decreased temperature at baseline
Fluids given in large volumes should be warmed
Consider the temperature and volume of surgical irrigation and tumescent solutions
Mood stabilizers such as lithium may interact with benzodiazepines causing hypothermia
Hypothyroidism

Box 10.12 *Continued*
Hyperthermia
Rare in the operating room, but may indicate serious process
Infection
Increased metabolic rate
Pheochromocytoma
Hyperthyroidism
Neuroleptic malignant syndrome
Malignant hyperthermia (see Box 10.13)

Box 10.13

Although outside the scope of this discussion, malignant hypothermia must be considered in the immediate differential diagnosis any time a patient has received succinylcholine or volatile anesthetics.
Key points in treatment include the following:

• Stopping the triggering agent
• Hyperventilation with 100% FIO_2
• Cooling the patient
• Providing supportive care
• Volume expansion
• Dantrolene therapy

(MHAUS, the Malignant Hyperthermia Association of the United States staffs a telephone hotline for consultation 24 hours a day at (800) MHHYPER.)

Temperature monitoring should be employed for all general anesthetics. Prevention of hypothermia and detection of the rare but catastrophic complication of malignant hyperthermia are the most important indications for temperature monitoring. General and neuraxial anesthetics promote vasodilatation speeding heat loss. Cold ambient air temperature, evaporative losses, instillation of cold fluids, and surgical exposure all further contribute to heat

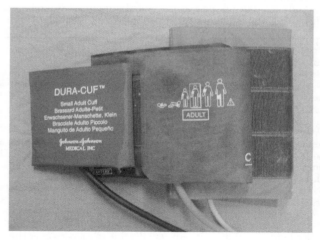

Figure 10.6. Blood pressure cuff.

loss. Hypothermia is associated with decreased metabolic rate; however, shivering in the postoperative period raises metabolic rate and oxygen demand, and has been associated with ischemia and postoperative myocardial infarction. Temperature monitoring allows the anesthesiologist to adjust the patient's microclimate by warming fluids, using passive or active warmers, and controlling room temperature to maintain a state of normothermia (see Box 10.14). Temperature probe location should approximate core body temperature. In the anesthetized patient, esophageal, nasal, rectal, or bladder probes are easily placed. In the awake patient, the best alternative may be a transcutaneous or axillary probe.

Box 10.14

Techniques to Maintain Normothermia
Adjust ambient temperature
Minimize exposure, using warmed blankets if possible
Humidify inhaled gases
Warm infusions, irrigation, and tumescent solutions
Employ active warming devices

In addition to monitoring temperature, the anesthesiologist must also be able to take steps to maintain the patient's temperature. For short duration cases with limited surgical exposure, simply keeping the patient covered may be sufficient. For cases of longer duration, a fluid warmer or forced hot air warmer may be required. Commercial warming systems are available with upper body, lower body, and under patient "blankets" that bathe the patient in warm air.

Malignant hyperthermia, a rare inherited disorder of increased skeletal muscle metabolism, may be induced by succinylcholine or volatile anesthetics. It presents as increased temperature, end-tidal CO_2, skeletal muscle rigidity, and tachycardia. Treatment involves removal of inciting agent, cooling, and dantrolene sodium. Dantrolene may be of specific interest to office-based practitioners, because it is often a weak point in the available pharmacy (see Box 10.15). Owing to its relatively high cost and short shelf life (3 years from date of manufacture), many facilities may be reluctant to incur the cost (approximately $2,700 for the recommended supply of 36 vials) associated with maintaining an adequate supply.

Box 10.15

Dantrolene Dosing
Provided as a sterile powder, dantrolene must be reconstituted in sterile water (60 mL vial). Initial bolus dose is 2.5 mg per kg IV. Dose may repeated every 5 minutes to a total dose of 10 mg per kg.

TECHNOLOGY AND OFFICE-BASED ANESTHESIA

The topics of awareness and depth of anesthesia are frequently appearing in both scholarly and lay publications. Awareness under anesthesia is an uncommon event often quoted to occur in 0.1% to 0.2% of anesthetics. Although rare, the psychological effects of intraoperative awareness may be devastating, leading to post-traumatic stress disorder and prolonged morbidity. Several clinical situations predispose a patient to awareness, including trauma, cardiac surgery, and obstetric emergency. In these situations, it is questionable whether monitoring of awareness would reduce the incidence of recall, as the light anesthetic plane is usually due to concern over the patient's inability to tolerate the hemodynamic effects of a deeper anesthetic plane.

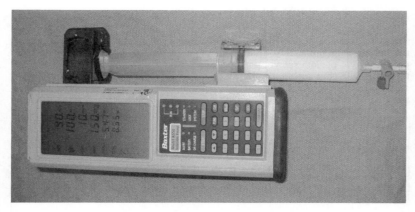

Figure 10.7. Programmable infusion pump set to deliver propofol.

Currently available devices attempt to ascertain depth of anesthesia by monitoring and processing the electroencephalogram. Several proprietary devices are available in the market and are currently being studied in an effort to determine efficacy. Depth of anesthesia/awareness monitoring may provide several benefits to the office-based provider. The ability to accurately monitor anesthetic depth may allow for decreased use of anesthetic agents, allow for more rapid recovery, prevent overmedication, minimize untoward effects, and increase turnover and efficiency. At present, these devices should be considered as a useful tool and when coupled with other available information can assist in tailoring the depth of anesthesia to individual patient requirements.

Automated charting systems are currently in widespread use, freeing the practitioner from charting vital signs and allowing more time for patient care. These systems can be linked to the anesthesia machine and have the ability to record both inspired and expired agent, oxygen, and CO_2 concentrations. Software may be customized to allow for point and click charting, saving additional time. Although these devices may save time and improve accuracy of charting, they are costly to install and maintain.

Currently available infusion pumps allow for precise administration of intravenous medications, and allow for quick titration and adjustment of dose. The next generation machine will likely allow for programmable bolus dosing and variable rate infusions (see Figure. 10.7).

CONCLUSIONS

The office-based environment provides for increased patient comfort, satisfaction, and convenience. Preoperative evaluation and screening is essential to ensure patients are appropriate for planned procedures and comorbidities recognized. Although most cases in the office setting involve healthy patients undergoing relatively minor procedures, the anesthesiologist must remain vigilant, prepare for, and be able to respond to complications that may develop (see Box 10.16). Responsibility for ensuring the physical plant is adequately equipped and maintained falls to the anesthesiologist. Additional responsibilities include the development of contingency plans and transfer policies in the event of a patient requiring more care than can be given in the office setting. Establishment of procedures and protocols for recovering patients as well as supervising a recovery area and staff development may also fall to the office-based anesthesia provider. Office-based anesthesia provides many unique challenges to the anesthesiologist. In the office setting, the anesthesiologist leaves behind the support systems found in the hospital setting and must rely upon himself or herself to provide all aspects of preoperative, perioperative, postoperative, and emergency care. It is crucial to remember that although the office-based environment may allow for increased patient comfort, satisfaction, convenience, and privacy, safety should always come first.

Box 10.16

The best monitor is a vigilant anesthesia provider.
The primary goal of the anesthesia provider is a safe anesthetic.

A backup oxygen supply, a means of positive pressure ventilation, a defibrillator, and an adequate emergency pharmacy should be available.
A formal plan for transfer of patients requiring increased level of care must be in place.

SUGGESTED READINGS

American Heart Association. 2005 American Heart Association guidelines for cardiopulmonary resuscitation and emergency cardiovascular care. *Circulation*. 2005;112(suppl): IV1–IV205. http://circ.ahajournals.org/content/vol112/24_suppl/#. Last accessed November 2006.

American Heart Association. Highlights of the 2005 American Heart Association guidelines for cardiopulmonary resuscitation and emergency cardiovascular care. *Curr Emerg Cardiovasc Care*. 2005;16: 1–22.

American Society of Anesthesiologists. *Standards for basic anesthetic monitoring*. October 25, 2005. http://www.asahq.org/publicationsAndServices/standards/02.pdf. Last accessed November 2006.

MHAUS. *What is malignant hypothermia?* Last updated 8/31/04. http://www.mhaus.org/index.cfm/fuseaction/OnlineBrochures.Display/BrochurePK/8AABF3FB-13B0-430F-BE20FB32516B02D6.cfm. Last accessed November 2006.

Surgical Procedures in the Office-Based Setting

D. Jonathan Bernardini and Fred E. Shapiro

With the recent advances in modern medicine and medical technology, an increasing number of physicians are able to perform more advanced and complex surgical procedures in their offices. Although the list of these procedures continues to grow everyday, most of the surgical procedures performed in a doctor's office involve some form of sedation and analgesia in order to lessen the pain and anxiety of the surgery. Regardless of whether it is a simple mole removal, breast augmentation and reduction, liposuction, hernia repair, or knee arthroscopy, a rapidly growing number of patients prefer to have these surgeries performed in a doctor's office rather than in hospitals or ambulatory surgical centers. As we saw in Chapter 2, patients and surgeons make their choices based on issues of cost, convenience, and scheduling. When one looks at the statistics, it appears that over the next few years more complex procedures are likely to become commonplace. Indeed, some office-based procedures are of such degree of complexity that they involve general anesthesia (GA) to provide a total loss of consciousness in the surgical patient (1). This becomes an added burden to all health care providers involved; the desire to keep up with the trends and advances, yet maintain the traditional standard of providing a safe, pleasant, and comfortable experience for the patient.

According to the American Society of Anesthesiologists' (ASA) *Guidelines for Office-Based Anesthesia*, it is estimated that in 2005, ten million procedures were performed in doctors' offices—twice the number of office-based surgeries performed in 1995. Furthermore, while 80% of surgeries are currently performed in hospitals or ambulatory surgical centers, we are seeing the same trend in the movement to the office-based setting as we saw 20 years ago with the shift from the inpatient to the outpatient setting. Currently, approximately one out of ten surgeries are performed in a doctor's office.

While it is nearly impossible to list the myriad surgical procedures performed in any number of subspecialist physician offices, this chapter will attempt to cover some of the more common procedures. Many of the

---

Box 11.1 • Standard Equipment

Noninvasive Monitoring Equipment
1. Blood pressure measuring device and cuff
2. Electrocardiogram (ECG)
3. Oxygen and gas analyzer
4. Capnography
5. Pulse oximeter
6. Temperature probe
7. Nerve stimulator

Standard Anesthesia Equipment
1. Airway equipment
2. Suction
3. Emergency drugs and "Code" cart
4. Anesthesia machine

Table 11.1. Recommended doses of commonly used drugs in the operating room

Drug	Bolus Dose	Infusion Rate
Sedatives/Anxiolytics/ Amnestics		
Lorazepam	0.02–0.08 mg/kg IV 0.05 mg/kg PO	
Midazolam	0.02–0.1 mg/kg IV 0.5–0.75 mg/kg PO	
Dexmedetomidine (α_2 agonist)	1 μg/kg IV over 10–15 min	0.2–0.7 μg/kg/h
Intravenous Anesthetics		
Propofol	2–2.5 mg/kg IV	25–200 μg/kg/min
Etomidate	0.2–0.6 mg/kg IV	
Methohexital	1–1.5 mg/kg IV (induction) 0.2–0.4 mg/kg IV (sedation)	20–60 μg/kg/min
Thiopental	3–5 mg/kg IV (induction) 0.5–1.5 mg/kg IV (sedation)	30–200 μg/kg/min
Ketamine	1–4 mg/kg IV (induction) 0.2–1 mg/kg IV (sedation)	10–75 μg/kg/min
Opiate Analgesics		
Fentanyl	0.25–1 μg/kg IV (25–100 μg/dose IV p.r.n.)	
Remifentanil	0.5–1 μg/kg IV	0.025–2 μg/kg/min
Sufentanil	0.5–30 μg/kg IV (10–50 μg IV p.r.n.)	0.3–1.5 μg/kg/h
Morphine	0.05–0.1 mg/kg IV	
Nonopiate Analgesics		
Ketorolac	15–30 mg IV	
Inhaled Anesthetics		
Nitrous oxide (inspired concentration)	30%–70%	
Desflurane (MAC)	6.0	
Sevoflurane (MAC)	2.05	
Muscle Relaxants		
Succinylcholine	1–1.5 mg/kg IV (intubation)	
Cisatracurium	0.15–0.2 mg/kg IV (intubation) 0.03 mg/kg IV (maintenance)	
Rocuronium	0.6–1.2 mg/kg IV (RSI)	
Vecuronium	0.1 mg/kg IV (intubation) 0.01–0.02 mg/kg IV (maintenance)	

Table 11.1. (*Continued*)

Drug	Bolus Dose	Infusion Rate
Reversal Agents		
Edrophonium (with atropine)	0.5–1.0 mg/kg IV	
Neostigmine (with glycopyrrolate)	0.07 mg/kg IV, 5 mg max	
Anticholinergics		
Atropine	10–15 μg/kg	
Glycopyrrolate	7–10 μg/kg	
Antiemetics		
Dolasetron	12.5 mg IV	
Ondansetron	0.1 mg/kg IV, 4 mg max	

MAC, monitored anesthesia care; RSI, rapid sequence induction.
Modified from: Sa Rego MM, Mehernoor FW, White PF. The changing role of monitored anesthesia care in the ambulatory setting. *Anesth Analg.* 1997;85:1020–1036, (2).

office-based procedures would benefit equally from the available methods of anesthesia (i.e., local, regional, monitored anesthesia care [MAC], GA—see Chapter 7) and will vary from patient to patient depending on a number of situations and variables.

With office-based surgical procedures, as with hospital or ambulatory surgical center–based procedures, patients will need to undergo a detailed history and physical examination. All comorbidities, medications, including over-the-counter and herbal preparations, allergies, problems with previous anesthesia, and psychosocial details will need to be factored into the anesthetic plan. Finally, the anesthesiologist may decide that a patient's comorbidities and other factors preclude him from a surgical procedure in an office setting.

When the decision has been made to proceed in the office setting, it is crucial to insure that all necessary monitors, airway adjuncts, anesthesia equipment, and other devices are present and that they are in good operating condition *before* beginning a procedure where any type of sedation or anesthesia will be administered.

Table 11.1 and Box 11.1 are essential items for the office-based setting. A comprehensive list can be found in Chapter 10. There will be individual variations based on the specific procedure, the facility, and the type of anesthesia planned.

COMMON COSMETIC SURGICAL PROCEDURES

The section that follows discusses the *seven* most common cosmetic surgical procedures including their anesthetic considerations and complications (see Box 11.2).

Box 11.2 • The Top Seven Cosmetic Surgical Procedures

1. Liposuction
2. Augmentation mammoplasty
3. Reduction mammoplasty
4. Blepharoplasty

> **Box 11.2   *Continued***
> 5. Rhinoplasty
> 6. Rhytidectomy
> 7. Hair transplantation

Liposuction

Liposuction is the most common cosmetic operation performed in the United States. It is the surgical removal of subcutaneous fat by means of aspiration cannulas, introduced through small skin incisions, assisted by suction. It is also referred to as liposuction surgery, suction-assisted lipectomy, suction lipoplasty, fat suction, blunt suction lipectomy, and liposculpture (3).

Procedure

The original technique developed in the 1970s has been modified and over the last decade has been enhanced by the subcutaneous infusion of crystalloid fluid containing local anesthetic and epinephrine. The resulting mixture of fat and infused wetting solution is aspirated through cannulas. Wetting solutions typically consist of 1 L (=1,000 mL) of Ringer's lactate containing 0.25 to 1 mg of epinephrine and 200 to 1,000 mg of lidocaine (4,5). A concentration of epinephrine of 1 per 1,000,000 (1 mg/1 L) provides excellent vasoconstriction after 10 to 20 minutes before aspiration of the adipose tissue. The amount of lidocaine used depends primarily on the mode of anesthesia. Lower concentrations of lidocaine will provide adequate postoperative analgesia and can be used for patients receiving GA or regional anesthesia. Higher concentrations of lidocaine are used for patients undergoing local or MAC anesthesia. The choice of anesthetic depends on the surgical region, the extent of adipose resection, the length of the procedure, and patient preference (5).

Typically, 1 mL of wetting solution will be used for each 1 mL of anticipated adipose resection. More dramatic results can be achieved with large-volume liposuction (>5,000 mL) whereas more subtle results are achieved with small-volume liposuction (<5,000 mL) (5). Tumescent liposuction involves a fluid infusion of two to three times the volume of the anticipated adipose resection. This is a method of performing liposuction under *local anesthesia* and precludes the use of additional anesthetic medications at dosages that may cause loss of airway reflexes or suppression of respiratory drive (3).

More recent developments involve the use of ultrasound assisted liposuction (UAL) in which ultrasound waves are targeted on the area to be treated, and fat cells are disrupted which can then be removed in a similar manner as the Illouz technique. This is a technique that will be used in conjunction with conventional liposuction more frequently in the future.

The procedure may take 2 to 7 hours depending on the extent of surgical resection. Large-volume procedures may require postoperative hospitalization for patient monitoring and pain control. Pain is managed immediately following surgery with the use of intravenous narcotics followed by oral analgesics as an inpatient and after discharge. The area treated will be wrapped with compression dressings to minimize swelling and bruising, although moderate to severe bruising is not uncommon, especially in the first several postoperative days. Patients are encouraged to ambulate on the day following surgery, progressively increasing to regularly walking after 2 weeks with full resumption of activities after a minimum of 4 weeks.

Anesthetic Considerations

It is important to recognize that liposuction is not a trivial procedure; a clear and detailed medical history and physical examination are required to insure safe treatment and a successful outcome. Certain physical signs will guide the surgeon and anesthesiologist in the assessment and suitability for surgery. Particular areas of the body should be approached with caution, notably the areas around the lower part of the buttock and the inner, outer, and posterior aspects of the thigh because of the risk of complications and contouring deformities.

Ideally, patients considering liposuction should be ASA category I or II, physically active, and have maintained a stable weight for 6 months to 1 year. The procedural techniques described in the preceding text have been developed to reduce blood loss and provide adequate postoperative analgesia. Intravenous fluids should be limited when performing large-volume procedures due to the large volumes of wetting solution utilized. Approximately two thirds of the wetting solution injected subcutaneously will be absorbed into the intravascular space. Conversely, larger volumes of intravenous fluids are required for small-volume liposuction to augment the small volumes of wetting solution (5).

Anesthetic Technique

In small-volume liposuction, adequate pain relief may be provided by the anesthetic infiltrate solutions alone or with a combination of local anesthetic and varying degrees of sedation. Large-volume cases typically require regional (spinal, epidural) or GA. Regional anesthesia has raised some concern regarding the associated vasodilation and the resulting potential for increased blood loss and fat embolization. GA allows for larger adipose resections and for the procedure to be done in all body regions while providing a greater degree of patient comfort (5).

Table 11.2 includes examples of typical general and MAC anesthetics for this and other appropriate surgical procedures (5).

Table 11.2.   Examples of typical general and monitored anesthesia care anesthetics

General Anesthesia	MAC Anesthesia

Premedication
    Midazolam 2 mg IV (in holding area)
Induction
    Propofol 2.0–2.5 mg/kg IV or
    Thiopental 3–5 mg/kg IV or
    ± Fentanyl 1 μg/kg IV
Muscle Relaxation
    Succinylcholine 1 mg/kg IV (for
        intubation)
    Vecuronium 0.1 mg/kg IV or
    Cisatracurium 0.2 mg/kg IV or
    Rocuronium 0.6–1.2 mg/kg IV or
Maintenance of Anesthesia
    O_2 30%–100%
    ± N_2O 0%–70% plus
    Desflurane or sevoflurane
Reversal of muscle relaxation:
    Neostigmine 0.07 mg/kg IV plus
    Glycopyrrolate 0.01 mg/kg IV
Analgesia:
    Fentanyl 25 μg IV titrated to effect
        up to 100 μg total
	Midazolam 2 mg IV (in holding area)
	    and
	0.25–1 mg IV during procedure
	    titrated to effect
	O_2 3–4 L/min by nasal cannula or
	    6–8 L/min by face mask with
	    capnograph
	Propofol 1–1.5 mg/kg IV then
	    50–100 μg/kg/min or
	Dexmedetomidine 1 μg/kg for
	    15–20 min then 0.2–0.7 μg/kg/h or
	Remifentanil 0.25–0.75 μg/kg/min
	Fentanyl 12.5–25 μg IV can be
	    titrated to effect and monitor for
	    respiratory depression

Table 11.2.   (*Continued*)

General Anesthesia	MAC Anesthesia
Morphine 1–4 mg IV titrated to effect up to 8 mg total (Monitor for respiratory depression) Nausea prophylaxis Dolasetron 12.5 mg IV ± Metoclopramide 10 mg IV Consider OG tube placement and suction for patients at risk for postoperative nausea and vomiting (PONV). O_2 100% Suction oropharynx Extubate (based on standard extubation criteria)	

OG, orogastric.
Modified from: Jaffe RA, Samuels SI. *Anesthesiologist's manual of surgical procedures,* 3rd ed. Philadelphia: Lippincott Williams & Wilkins; 2004:114–137, 892–894, B1–B4.

For patients receiving GA, either an endotracheal tube (ETT) or laryngeal mask airway (LMA) can be used. Factors such as gastroesophageal reflux (GERD) and unusual patient positioning may preclude the use of an LMA. All patients should receive adequate intravenous access based on fluid requirements, anticipated blood loss, and potential for receiving blood products during the procedure. For most cosmetic surgery, an 18- or 20-gauge angio-catheter in either upper extremity should be sufficient, although each patient should be evaluated and managed independently.

Complication

Liposuction has the potential for complications from a number of different etiologies (see Box 11.3). Local anesthetic toxicity from the wetting solution is a concern; cardiac dysrhythmias and deaths related to this have been reported (6). Lidocaine dosages in the wetting solution of 35 to 55 mg per kg are generally accepted as safe and are routinely employed (3,4). Bupivacaine has not been studied for use in liposuction wetting solutions (5). Epinephrine doses should not exceed 0.07 mg per kg, although doses as high as 0.10 mg per kg have been used safely. Its use should be avoided in patients with pheochromocytoma, hyperthyroidism, severe hypertension, cardiac disease, and peripheral vascular disease (5).

Box 11.3 • Complications of Liposuction

Hypervolemia
Hypovolemia

Lidocaine toxicity
Pulmonary embolism
Hypothermia

Owing to the potentially large volumes of fluid utilized during this procedure, the potential for volume overload exists which can lead to heart failure and cardiogenic pulmonary edema. For example, the "tumescent technique" where 2 to 3 mL of wetting solution is infiltrated for every mL of anticipated lipoaspirate, leaves behind 50% to 70% of the infiltrated volume (5).

Conversely, large volume liposuction, in the absence of adequate fluid replacement, may result in moderate to severe hypovolemia and, possibly, shock. Although excessive blood loss was seen more commonly in the early days of liposuction before the use of tumescence, it continues to be of concern. Related to all of these concerns is the risk of hypothermia due to the large volumes of wetting solutions, which are not typically warmed. The rapid infusion of large volumes of relatively cold fluid can quickly lower body temperature to dangerous levels. Great care should be taken to vigorously maintain the patient's body temperature using heated forced-air units and intravenous fluid warmers. Other complications include pulmonary embolism, fat emboli, peripheral nerve injury, and abdominal cavity perforation (5).

Longer-term risks are related to decreased mobility, particularly if surgery involved the legs or lower abdomen. The patient is at increased risk of developing a deep venous thrombosis (DVT), so prophylactic treatment of this condition may be necessary.

Finally, as is the case with all surgical procedures, there may be postoperative inflammation or infection resulting from tissue trauma. Preincisional prophylactic antibiotics are routinely used and greatly reduce these risks.

Augmentation Mammoplasty

There is documentation of an attempted breast augmentation performed in the late 19th century when a surgeon transplanted a lipoma from the back of a woman into her breasts. Various materials have been used over the years from liquid paraffin injections to gel implants to the permanent tissue expanders in current use.

Although implants have been used in surgical practice since the 1960s, problems associated with silicone gel implants resulted in a moratorium on their use issued from the U.S. Food and Drug Administration (FDA) in 1991 for routine cosmetic procedures, resulting in surgeons looking for an alternative material. Although saline-filled implants proved a safer alternative, problems with leaks led to their falling out of favor. Many surgeons preferred the longevity and appearance of the silicone gel implant. In April 2005, the FDA advisory panel made a recommendation to allow one of two silicone breast implant manufacturers to market implants in the US market after the 13-year ban.

Experience has taught us that these types of implants have the best possible effect when placed beneath the muscle layer of the chest wall. Modern surgery involves the placement of an implant that may then be expanded periodically by sequential injections of saline from a reservoir directly into it, until the desired effect is achieved.

Procedure

Breast implants are placed through skin incisions made at various sites. An inframammary incision is the most common site, involving a 3 to 4 cm incision in the inframammary crease. Alternative locations include periareolar, transaxillary, or periumbilical.

Placing the implant beneath the breast but above the pectoralis or beneath the pectoralis muscle under the breast will be a decision made by the surgeon based on his or her experience and the preference of the patient. Disadvantages of submuscular placement include increased postoperative pain, limitation on size of implant, and the potential for lateral movement of implant. Advantages include reduced sensory changes around the nipple, less bleeding, reduced capsular contracture, and ease of interpretation of mammographic studies later in life.

The procedure typically takes 1 to 3 hours to complete and the breasts are typically bandaged to help reduce inflammation and bruising. Postoperative analgesia is usually achieved with intravenous opiates and patient controlled analgesia (PCA), if hospitalized, with transition to oral narcotic analgesics. Most patients are discharged home on the day of surgery unless there are pre-existing medical conditions or postoperative pain issues that require greater attention, in which case the patient may be admitted.

Anesthetic Technique

Breast augmentation is typically performed under GA. This procedure can also be performed using local anesthesia in combination with sedation or an MAC anesthetic, although this is not very common (Table 11.2).

Complications

The most common problem associated with breast implants is capsular contracture. This is a result of the tissues around the implant scarring and contracting. This puts pressure on the soft implant and may distort it and cause pain.

Because of the frequent position changes from supine to upright and the subsequent changes in lung pressures as well as the proximity of the surgical procedure to the chest wall, pneumothorax is a potential risk of breast surgery. As with all surgical procedures there is a risk of bleeding and infection. Excessive bleeding may require reoperation and infection may require the implant to be removed and reinserted once the infection has been treated.

Reduction Mammoplasty

Many women are genetically predisposed to macromastia and the condition may be aggravated by weight gain or hormonal influences such as pregnancy. Techniques of breast reduction have been developed over the last 100 years for both aesthetic and functional purposes. A cycle of increasing size and weight placing increasing stress on suspensory breast ligaments results in progressive descent of the breast.

Procedure

Numerous techniques are recognized for breast reduction; broadly, they may be divided into removal of breast tissue with pedicle formation or, less commonly, liposuction alone. When the breast becomes very large, it is typical to remove large quantities of tissue leaving a pedicle that provides an adequate blood supply. If the breast is not overly pendulous or large and the skin has retained its elasticity, then liposuction alone may be utilized. Liposuction in the breast enables minimal scarring but may result in sensory nerve damage.

The patient will be marked to define the new site of the nipple once breast tissue has been removed. Excess tissue is removed and the process of reshaping the existing breast occurs. It is vital to keep a good blood supply to surviving skin and breast tissue. This procedure may take 1 to 2 hours per breast depending on the extent of the reduction. Patients can be discharged on the day of surgery or remain in the hospital overnight, especially if postoperative analgesia is of concern.

After the operation, the breasts will be bandaged to minimize inflammation and bruising. Pain control will be administered as required. Drains may have been placed at the time of the operation to collect any buildup of blood or inflammatory fluid. These are usually removed after 1 day. Patient followup usually happens after 2 weeks, again at 3 months then finally at 6 months, when swelling should have resolved. It may take a year or longer for the final appearance to be evident.

Anesthetic Technique

Breast reduction mammoplasty is typically performed under GA preceded by mild sedation and/or an anxiolytic (Table 11.2).

Complications

A major complication of this procedure is damage to the nipple and compromise of its blood supply. Other complications include bleeding, accumulation of inflammatory fluids leading to seroma, and infection. Reoperation is rare and most people are able to resume normal activities within 1 month of surgery.

Blepharoplasty (Eyelid Lift)

People have had eyelid surgery for over a 100 years but it has been in the last 20 that significant improvements have been made both in terms of the understanding of the underlying conditions and their successful treatment. Planning the procedure will involve deciding how much skin and fat will need to be removed and determining the site of the lachrymal gland that may need to be repositioned.

Procedure

The procedure itself will last approximately 1 to 3 hours depending on the extent of work required. If one is having all four eyelids done, the surgeon will probably work on the upper lids first, then the lower ones.

Typically, the surgeon will make incisions following the natural lines of the eyelids; in the creases of the upper lids, and just below the lashes in the lower lids. The incisions may extend into the outer corners of the eyes. The surgeon separates the skin from underlying fatty tissue and muscle, removes excess fat, and often trims sagging skin and muscle. The incisions are then closed with very fine sutures.

If there is a pocket of fat beneath the lower eyelids without necessitating skin removal, the surgeon may perform a transconjunctival blepharoplasty. In this procedure the incision is made inside the lower eyelid, leaving no visible scar. It is usually performed on younger patients with thicker, more elastic skin.

After the operation, the eyes will be lubricated and bandaged. The patient can expect swelling and bruising in the first 24 hours; cold packs are usually applied to the face to minimize inflammation. The patient is typically discharged home on the day of surgery.

Anesthetic Technique

Blepharoplasty is usually performed under local anesthesia in conjunction with MAC (Table 11.2). Please refer to the discussion in the section on Rhytidectomy (Face Lift) regarding the use of DEX during TIVA in aesthetic facial surgery.

Complications

The most serious complication of surgery involving the eye is blindness, although this is very rare occurrence, with a reported incidence of 0.04% (8). This may be due to bleeding within and behind the eye, causing pressure on the optic nerve and its blood supply. Should this happen it will require immediate attention and further surgery. Postoperative ectropion can occur if overexcision of skin from the lower eyelid occurs (5). Corneal abrasions may also occur and require an ophthalmology consult. Treatment is usually use of ointment and time for healing. Other complications include infection at the operative site, abscess formation around the sutures, excessive swelling, or bleeding. Furthermore, eyes may become very dry, the lower eyelids may be pulled down, or an ectropion may develop.

Rhinoplasty

This is one of the oldest known reconstructive plastic surgery procedures, with historic records dating back to Egyptian times of people with nasal deformities undergoing corrective treatment.

Modern day rhinoplasty encompasses a wide range of surgical procedures on the nose used to improve both function and appearance. There are two main approaches: open and closed rhinoplasty. Open surgery involves both internal and external incisions whereas closed techniques rely on internal incisions only. It has been suggested that closed techniques involve shorter operative time, less dissection, minimize scarring and inflammation, and help the patient recover more quickly.

Procedure

The surgery will usually take 1 to 2 hours and the surgeon will decide how best to refashion the nose, from work on the septum to sculpting the tip. Should extensive work be required, because this is almost always necessary, an osteotomy may be performed involving a controlled fracture through certain bony nasal components.

After the operation, significant swelling and bruising will likely occur. A splint will be applied to help the nose maintain its new shape. Nasal packs or soft plastic splints may also be placed in the nostrils to stabilize the septum, the dividing wall between the air passages.

The patient may notice that the swelling and bruising around the eyes will increase at first, reaching a peak after 2 or 3 days. Applying cold compresses will reduce this swelling. Most of the swelling and bruising should resolve within 2 weeks. Patients are discharged home on the day of surgery.

Anesthetic Technique

Rhinoplasty can be performed under local or GA, depending on the extent of the procedure. With GA, oropharyngeal packing is typically placed after intubation of the patient to prevent blood from draining into the esophagus. Furthermore, an orogastric tube should be placed to suction any blood or other fluids from the patient's stomach in an attempt to avoid postoperative vomiting; the orogastric tube should be removed before patient emergence. With local anesthesia and sedation/MAC, because the gag reflex is intact, no oropharyngeal packing is placed (Table 11.2).

Complications

The main complications relate to bleeding that may obstruct the nose or significant facial swelling. Preoperative education should be offered about specific activities which one should try to refrain from such as coughing, sneezing, or any maneuver that could raise one's blood pressure because these may provoke both bleeding and inflammation. It may be necessary to have emotional support because this type of surgery has profound visual impact and usually requires a few weeks for recovery. In some cases further surgery may be necessary. Other complications include infections, stitch abscesses, and ongoing postoperative pain.

Rhytidectomy (Facelift)

Forehead lifts date back to the early 20th century; however, as with most plastic surgical procedures the last 20 or 30 years has seen tremendous advances in a variety of techniques. A facelift may provide one of the most dramatic effects in cosmetic plastic surgery.

Procedure

Although surgeons will plan and perform the procedure in their own way, it usually begins with administration of lidocaine in combination with epinephrine. These are injected subcutaneously to anesthetize the area of surgery, decrease the amount of bleeding, and help to elevate the skin above the underlying muscle layer. The procedure may also be performed under intravenous sedation depending on the preference of the patient, surgeon, and anesthetist. Incisions are usually made around the hairline at the temple and continued around the upper part of the ear, extending as far as the ear lobe or lower in certain cases.

The surgeon will need to separate the skin from the underlying fat and muscle layers. The underlying muscle will be stretched and excess fat may be removed. Once the surgeon is satisfied with the desired result, the various tissue layers will be sutured. The skin incision may be closed either with sutures or small metal clips. A small drain may be placed to prevent accumulation of fluid and an antibiotic ointment may be applied to the sutured skin followed by bandaging to minimize swelling.

Most patients are discharged home either on the day of the surgery or, if necessary, the following day. One should expect some soreness, bruising, and inflammation. This will take a few weeks to finally resolve. In the meantime iced compresses for the first 48 hours may help to decrease bruising and swelling. Most patients will require oral analgesics for pain. Postoperative swelling, particularly around the eyes, is common.

Anesthetic Technique

In the past, it was commonplace for a rhytidectomy to be performed under GA. However, with the advances in safe short-acting anesthetic agents and patient education combined with a greater number of procedures performed in the office-based setting, many patients request the following:

- Sedation
- Relief from anxiety
- To be unaware of what is happening (during the procedure)
- To be pain free
- No postoperative nausea and vomiting (PONV)
- Not to have an ETT or "GA"

At Beth Israel Deaconess Medical Center, we use a total intravenous anesthesia (TIVA) technique using dexmedetomidine (DEX) in combination with propofol, ketamine, and midazolam. This technique utilizes a combination of sedation, anxiolysis, and non-narcotic analgesia.

DEX is in the α_2 agonist class of drugs. It has sedative, analgesic, and anxiolytic properties and reduces the requirements for other sedatives and analgesics in the intraoperative and postoperative periods. It is a drug that fits perfectly with the "fast track" philosophy.

The key issue that led to our routine use of DEX in aesthetic facial surgery is the added *safety* to the patients. The cardiorespiratory effects of DEX combine intravenous sedation while allowing the patient to breathe room air spontaneously without the requirement of supplemental oxygen. This *avoids* the risk of combustion seen with the combination of oxygen and electrocautery/laser that is commonly used in outpatient surgery.

Recently, we performed a retrospective study evaluating 170 patients who received intravenous sedation with DEX. DEX appears to be a safe and effective anesthetic for patients undergoing aesthetic facial surgery. Based on the forthcoming studies, we hope to provide evidence to support the routine use of DEX in the outpatient setting. The following is a summary of the technique:

- Midazolam 2 to 4 mg IV in the holding area; an additional 2 to 4 mg IV can be given in the operating room (OR).

- All IV anesthetics and analgesics are diluted to a base of "10": 10 μg per mL (DEX, fentanyl) or 10 mg per mL (propofol, ketamine).
- Once in the OR, while the ASA standard monitors are being placed, loading doses of DEX (1 μg/kg) and ketamine (0.25–0.75 mg/kg) over 10 to 15 minutes are started.
- A urinary catheter is placed at the completion of the loading dose; the lack of movement or verbal response during urinary catheter placement is a good indication that an adequate level of sedation has been achieved for the forthcoming facial injection of local anesthetic.
- A DEX infusion is continued at 0.2 to 0.7 μg/kg/hour and a ketamine infusion is continued at 10 to 50 μg/kg/minute.
- A propofol infusion of 10 to 30 μg/kg/minute is started during the sterile preparation and drape and titrated based on the patient's response to the injection of local anesthetic into the desired surgical area.
- If the patient is unable to tolerate the local anesthetic injection, 1 to 2 mL of DEX (10 μg/mL) and 1 to 2 mL of ketamine (10 mg/mL) are bolused.
- In refractory patients, 1 to 2 mL of fentanyl (10 μg/mL) can be given and titrated to the patient's respiratory rate.
- Midazolam 1 to 2 mg IV every 1 to 2 hours can be given to maintain amnesia.
- The patient typically undergoes this anesthetic without supplemental oxygen. In the event of desaturation, the surgeon is asked to hold the electrocautery, and to perform a jaw-thrust maneuver. If the oxygen desaturation remains, supplemental oxygen is then administered by the anesthesia personnel through a face mask.
- At the conclusion of the case, all infusions are stopped when the surgical dressings are being placed. The patient is usually alert within 5 to 10 minutes and is able to move by themselves to the transport bed.

Refer to the discussion in the preceding text regarding the use of DEX during TIVA for aesthetic facial surgery (7).

Complications

From a surgical point of view, this procedure is typically not associated with many complications. Because of the extensive vascular supply to the face, bleeding with subsequent hematoma formation does rarely occur. There may be numbness of the face that usually resolves, bleeding early on that usually resolves spontaneously, and, finally, swelling and bruising in the early postoperative course. Although the patient may return to work activities within a week of the procedure, it is not recommended to engage in strenuous activity for a couple of weeks.

For the anesthesiologist, systemic toxicity from local anesthetic can be minimized by maintaining the dose of lidocaine at or below 5 mg per kg (7 mg/kg with epinephrine). A great deal of local anesthetic uptake can occur due to the vascularity of the face.

Hair Transplantation

Hair transplantation as a common procedure began in the 1960s with the work of Orentreich, a dermatologist. With a wide range of solutions claiming to restore hair growth or prevent its further demise are on the market, the definitive treatment remains surgical implantation. Although many believe hair loss (alopecia) to be a male phenomenon, approximately 15 million women in the United States suffer alongside 40 million men.

A significant factor in alopecia is the conversion of testosterone to dihydrotestosterone. Some individuals have autoimmune conditions resulting in extensive hair loss.

In planning treatment, the extent of hair loss is determined and the patient scored on the Hamilton pattern. Those with the greatest area of hair loss are not the best candidates because the most natural result is gained in those with limited loss. Medical therapy involves the use of minoxidil topical solutions and finasteride tablets.

Procedure

Hair transplantation involves the selection of a donor area on the patient's scalp from which hair may be taken, known as *minigrafts* and *micrografts*. Hair grafts range from a strip of hair containing up to 50 hairs to the smallest micrografts that may comprise individual hairs. The real difference between the types is the end result. The most natural looking result is derived from harvesting individual hairs and implanting them one at a time.

Once a donor site on the body has been identified, the hair is trimmed to allow ease of access to the hair and its follicle. A "punch graft" involving a round punch of the scalp and hair or a strip of hair may be harvested. The site of hair removal may require a small stitch to allow the skin to heal quickly. Once ready for transplantation, grafts are introduced in a progressive manner to the area to be treated. Because hair transplantation takes time, this process usually requires multiple treatments occurring over weeks or months depending on the size of the area being treated. Grafts are placed approximately an eight of an inch from one another in order to preserve scalp blood supply. Knowledge of the distribution of cutaneous sensory nerves of the scalp will assist the surgeon to adequately anesthetize the area to be treated.

A larger procedure involves raising a flap from an area of the scalp that is well covered by hair. Once the donor site has been identified, without damaging its blood supply, the flap can be rotated around to cover the bald area. Alternatively an area of baldness can be dealt with by excision of that region of scalp. These two methods are not suitable for everyone but have the advantage of achieving their results rapidly.

Complications

Hair transplantation is a low-risk surgical procedure, provided the patient has no underlying bleeding disorder or known reaction to local. Excess use of local anesthetic over the course of a long procedure can lead to local anesthetic toxicity, which can cause serious neurologic and cardiac complications. Pain may be treated with oral medication as required.

Anesthetic Technique

The most common anesthetic technique for hair transplantation procedures is the use of local anesthetics. Anxiolysis can be achieved with midazolam 0.5 to 2 mg IV several minutes before beginning the procedure or lorazepam 1 to 2 mg PO 1 hour preoperatively.

NONSURGICAL COSMETIC PROCEDURES

In 2005, the American Society of Aesthetic Plastic Surgeons (ASAPS) estimated that 12.5 million surgical and nonsurgical cosmetic procedures were performed in the United States; 75% of those were nonsurgical. With the growing interest in the office-based setting and the exponential rate of their growth, the most common cosmetic nonsurgical procedures are listed (see Box 11.4). To ensure patient safety, regardless of where the procedure is performed, if any anesthesia is utilized we recommend strict adherence to ASA standards for the anesthetic preparation, patient monitoring, and technique as noted in Tables 11.1 and 11.2 and Boxes 11.1 and 11.2 (and see Chapter 5).

Box 11.4 • The Most Common Cosmetic Nonsurgical Procedures

Dermabrasion
  Mechanical dermabrasion
  Laser dermabrasion
  Microdermabrasion
Chemical peels

Personnel who are familiar with and skilled in the administration of sedatives, anxiolytics, intravenous analgesics, and airway management, should be present for the entirety of these surgical procedures. In many cases, only small doses of sedatives and anxiolytics are being used, so the need for an anesthesiologist may be unnecessary and cost prohibitive. certified registered nurse anesthetists (CRNAs) and registered nurses (RNs) skilled in "conscious sedation techniques" are used in many settings for the administration of these medications and patient monitoring during procedures. In the overwhelming majority of states, CRNAs must work under the supervision of an anesthesiologist but in a few states or in rural or underserved areas, they are simply required to be under the supervision of a "physician." This typically refers to the surgeon who is performing the procedure. No matter what the specific regulations are, if higher doses of these medications are required, personnel skilled in emergency airway management, preferably those with formal anesthesia training, should be present during the entire surgical procedure.

Procedures

Dermabrasion

This technique, developed in New York in the 1950s by Abner Kurtin, is suitable for a variety of skin conditions. It is used mainly on the face because it is a visible area and the skin of the face has a high concentration of pilosebaceous glands that impact on the healing process. It is used in the treatment of acne scars and scarring due to traumatic injuries and surgical procedures. It may also be used to smooth areas of skin that are coarse. It is not a perfect cure because the skin is unlikely to look flawless; however particularly in the patient who has mild to moderate wrinkles and scarring, significant improvement will occur. The development of laser dermabrasion occurred in the 1980s and has become more popular in recent years.

It is important at the outset to identify accurately the patient's skin type. Commonly used is the Fitzpatrick classification from type I (always sun burns, fair skin) to type VI (never sun burns, black skin), or the Obagi classification which takes into account other factors, including skin thickness, firmness, fragility, and oiliness. On the basis of the skin type a treatment plan is proposed in the context of realistically attainable results and potential complications. Dark pigmented skin, in particular, is prone to developing hypertrophic scars. The risk of developing such a complication may outweigh the desired benefits.

Dermabrasion is contraindicated in certain conditions, namely collagen disorders, scleroderma, and cutis laxa, which may result in further scarring. Recent or ongoing use of isotretinoin, which damages the pilosebaceous glands that assist in the healing process, is also a contraindication. Previous radiation therapy to the site is also a relative contraindication.

Over the years, newer, more advanced techniques with potentially fewer risks of complications have been developed. Microdermabrasion uses tiny particles of aluminum oxide (comparable to fine sand), which are propelled onto the skin's surface and vacuumed up, taking with them dead skin cells.

Intense pulsed light (IPL) known as *photorejuvenation, lunchtime facelift, flash lamp facial*, and *FotoFacial*, uses rapid pulses of light that cause limited thermal damage to the lower layers of skin without disrupting the skin surface. It is aimed at permanent hair reduction, improving broken capillaries and spider veins and as a treatment for tightening the skin.

Light emitting diodes (LED), also known as *phototherapy*, is a light that is applied to the skin, delivering a stream of specific light wavelengths that pass through the top layers to the blood vessels and collagen. It is used to reduce fine lines and wrinkles, sun damage, acne, rosacea, eczema, and psoriasis. LED treatments are good in combination with chemical skin peels, microdermabrasion, and facials.

Microcurrent is a technology that uses a low-level electric current to manipulate facial muscles to improve underlying muscle tone. The microcurrent stimulates the circulation aiding collagen, elastin, and adenosine triphosphate (ATP) production. It may constitute an individual treatment or may be used in combination with microdermabrasion or IPL.

MECHANICAL DERMABRASION.   The area due to undergo dermabrasion is first clearly identified and marked. Anesthetic is infiltrated to the area and allowed to permeate. The surgeon then applies the handheld device across the skin, varying the depth and speed of the process. Initially there will be little or no bleeding; however, as further layers of skin are reached and removed, more bleeding points will become evident. It is not usually necessary to continue beyond that point and there will also be a greater risk of scar formation. Saline sponges soaked in epinephrine may be applied to decrease the bleeding areas.

At the end of the procedure a topical ointment will usually be applied to the abraded skin. The specific preparation varies between surgeons but it is petroleum based; topical antibiotics are usually avoided because they have a tendency to provoke inflammation. It is important to avoid direct sun exposure for a week—this is the length of time required for re-epithelialization of the skin to occur. It usually takes a few months before normal skin appearance is seen.

LASER DERMABRASION.   An alternative to a mechanical dermabrasion involves the use of a laser. Although early lasers in the 1980s used a continuous wave of energy, developments have led to pulsed lasers that have much fewer side effects, notably a smaller area of surrounding damage. Once again a formal examination and skin type assessment is made. A history of skin infections may require a course of treatment before the procedure. Active infections are a contraindication for this procedure. Laser dermabrasion is a more involved procedure beginning 4 to 6 weeks before with a course of daily cream applications that may include retinoic acid, hydroquinone, and α-hydroxy acid creams.

Following the procedure, the face is dressed with either a semiocclusive dressing that remains until the skin has healed or the application of an ointment directly to the skin. A course of oral antibiotics, antivirals, anti-inflammatories, and analgesics is usually prescribed. The skin should be treated as a second-degree burn so care is required both in washing and contact with sunlight. Depending on the depth of treatment, recovery may take several weeks. Patients can expect some fluid discharge and crusting over the sites of abrasion. Dressings are used until the superficial skin layers have re-epithelialized. The final effects of the procedure may take up to a year to be seen.

Chemical Peels

This procedure involves the application of chemicals to the skin, phenol or trichloroacetic acid, to produce a superficial burn. Once the tissue healing and re-epithelialization process is complete, the skin is smoother and firmer. Histologically, there are increased amounts of collagen and elastic fibers in the underlying dermis (8).

COMPLICATIONS. One of the greatest potential risks of these procedures is the development of an infection. These must be treated rapidly to avoid scarring. As mentioned earlier, there is also a risk of developing hypertrophic scars. If these develop, treatment with topical steroids, pressure bandages, or silicone dressings are used. Hyperpigmentation may also be a problem and can be treated with hydroquinones and bleaching agents. In addition, the patient may develop sensitive skin that is prone to inflammation when treated with other topical agents. Also, treated areas may become hypopigmented, particularly in darker individuals. Less common, but serious, complications include corneal injury due to insufficient eye protection during the procedure and the development of ectropion, particularly following repeated laser dermabrasion of the lower eyelid.

ANESTHETIC TECHNIQUE. A simple topical anesthetic with local anesthetic infiltration may suffice for some patients. A more commonly utilized technique is a regional block in the region of the face and neck together with some intravenous sedation. If necessary a patient may request a general anesthetic, although this is not common practice.

DENTAL PROCEDURES

According to the Society of Dental Anesthesiologists, most dental procedures performed in a dentist's office do not require the services of an anesthesiologist (see Box 11.5). Dentists are trained in the use of anxiolytics, sedatives, nitrous oxide, and airway management. However, depending on the specific needs of the patient or the complexity of the procedure, a deeper state of anesthesia may be required. Some patients simply prefer a higher level of anesthesia than others. Children, persons with "special needs," such as mental retardation, and those with a psychiatric condition, such as a dental phobia, may require a higher level of anesthesia. Local anesthesia is the most commonly used form of anesthesia in the dental office. Deep sedation and GA are used for complex procedures and for patients who have trouble controlling their movements or who feel they need a deeper level of anesthesia during treatment (9). To ensure patient safety, regardless of where the procedure is performed, if any anesthesia is utilized we recommend strict adherence to ASA standards for the anesthetic preparation, patient monitoring, and technique as shown in Tables 11.1 and 11.2 and Boxes 11.1 and 11.2.

Box 11.5 • The Most Common Dental Procedures

1. Fillings
2. Tooth restoration and replacement
3. Wisdom tooth extraction
4. Root canal therapy

Procedures

Dentists may recommend a procedure for one of several reasons, including prevention of tooth and gum disease, restoration of damaged or lost teeth, and cosmetic procedures to improve the appearance of one's teeth. Some of these procedures are straightforward, whereas others are more involved and, therefore, the complexity of the procedure and the accompanying anesthetic will vary (10).

Fillings

Teeth that have been affected by tooth decay (caries or cavities) require a filling. There are many different types of fillings, including metal alloys or amalgams, containing a combination of silver, tin, copper, and mercury, and composite resins. These are known as *direct fillings* and are placed directly into the cavity after the dentist has cleaned out the decay. Alternatives to restoring damaged or decayed teeth include porcelain veneers, crowns, and cast gold restorations and are known as *indirect fillings*. Dental amalgam is the best-known direct material. Cast gold alloy is the most durable indirect material. However, ceramics are gaining in popularity because of their longevity relative to other tooth-colored materials (5,11).

Anesthesia is typically administered by the dentist and includes a combination of topical and local anesthetics. Mild oral sedatives or anxiolytics may also be given.

Tooth Restoration and Replacement

When a tooth or a number of teeth are badly damaged or lost, they may be restored or replaced in a variety of ways including crowns, bridges, dentures, and dental implants. The decision on which method is utilized depends on the patient's health status and financial situation and insurance coverage.

Anesthesia is administered by the dentist and includes a combination of topical and local anesthetics. Mild oral sedatives or anxiolytics may also be given.

Wisdom Tooth Extraction

Also called *third molars*, wisdom teeth usually make their first appearance in young adults between the age of 15 and 25. Because most mouths are too small for these four additional molars, an extraction procedure, sometimes immediately after they surface, is often necessary. Most oral health specialists will recommend an immediate removal of the wisdom teeth, as early removal will help to eliminate problems, such as an impacted tooth that destroys the second molar. According to the American Academy of General Dentistry, third molar impaction is the most prevalent medical developmental disorder. Wisdom tooth extraction surgery involves removing the gum tissue that presides over the tooth, gently detaching the connective tissue between the tooth and the bone, removing the tooth, and suturing the opening in the gumline (5).

Anesthesia is administered by the dentist and includes a combination of topical and local anesthetics in conjunction with intravenous sedation and, possibly, inhaled nitrous oxide, a technique commonly referred to as *twilight sleep*. Some patients may require GA depending on the extent and complexity of the surgery and the particular needs of the patient (i.e., younger children, mentally retarded patients, and psychiatric patients).

Root Canal Therapy

Root canal therapy is designed to correct disorders of the dental pulp, the soft tissue around the tooth that contains nerves, blood vessels, and connective tissue. Teeth with abscessed nerves were once removed with corrective therapy. But now, in 95% of these cases of pulpal infection, the natural tooth can be saved through modern endodontic procedures. Without treatment, the infection of the dental pulp will spread to the bone around the tooth, making it unable to hold the tooth in place.

Treatment begins with the initial removal of the tooth crown to allow access to the pulpal tissue. Once the affected pulpal tissue is exposed, the affected area is removed. The area surrounding and containing the pulpal tissue is carefully cleaned, enlarged, and shaped to provide a clean, bondable surface for filling with a permanent filler to prohibit any further infection and discomfort. After filling, a crown is fabricated to complete the rescue and restoration of the natural tooth. The procedure is generally spread over several visits to assure that the infected pulp and associated bacteria have been adequately drained (5).

Anesthesia is administered by the dentist and includes a combination of topical and local anesthetics. Mild oral sedatives or anxiolytics may also be given. Again, based on the extent of the procedure and varying patient factors, choice of anesthetic technique may vary.

PODIATRY

Podiatric surgery can be performed in any of three commonly used locations—hospital OR, ambulatory surgery center, or office-based setting—depending on the patient's accompanying comorbidities. For instance, healthy patients can easily have their surgery in an ambulatory surgery center or office whereas very ill patients, many who are already hospitalized, will have their procedure performed in a hospital OR. To ensure patient safety, regardless of where the procedure is performed, if any anesthesia is utilized we recommend strict adherence to ASA standards for anesthetic preparation, patient monitoring, and technique as seen in Tables 11.1 and 11.2 and Boxes 11.1 and 11.2.

Procedures

There are many different podiatric surgeries that can be offered to patients. The more commonly offered procedures are listed in Box 11.6.

Box 11.6 • The Most Common Podiatric Procedures

1. Arthrodesis
2. Arthroereisis
3. Arthroplasty
4. Bone spur removal
5. Ganglion removal
6. Hallux limitus/rigidus
7. Bunion surgery
8. Haglund's deformity
9. Neuroma surgery
10. Plantar fasciitis
11. Tendon repair

Arthrodesis

Arthrodesis is the surgical fixation and fusion of a joint to relieve pain and provide support to the diseased joint. It is also known as *artificial ankylosis* or *syndesis*.

Arthroereisis

Arthroereisis (also called *arthrorisis* and *arthroerisis*) is defined as the limitation or restraint of excessive or abnormal motion across a joint. It is utilized for the treatment of symptomatic flexible flatfoot involving peritalar subluxation. In this procedure, an arthroereisis implant is placed to block the abnormal talar motion without damaging the subtalar joint or its function (12).

Arthroplasty

Arthroplasty is the surgical restoration of the integrity and functional power of a joint typically used in the repair of symptomatic "hammertoe."

Bone Spur Removal

A bone spur is an excessive growth of bone causing pain or limitation of movement. Spurs can develop at the edges of joints, tendons, and ligaments. Their removal can usually be undertaken under local anesthetic (13).

Ganglion Removal

Ganglions are benign soft tissue tumors of the joints and tendons. Symptomatic ganglions are removed by surgical excision.

Hallux Limitus/Rigidus

An arthritic condition of the big toe joint, it can cause pain and loss of motion by limiting or preventing dorsiflexion of the big toe while walking. The condition can be treated using a variety of surgical techniques, sometimes using artificial joints to treat the condition if the joint is beyond repair. These can be made of silastic rubber, titanium, or even ceramic (5).

Hallux Valgus (Bunion Surgery)

A painful enlargement of the joint situated at the base of the big toe. A bunion actually refers to the bony prominence or exostosis on the side of the big toe. A large sac of fluid, known as a *bursa*, can form over the enlarged joint that can then become inflamed and painful. Surgery involves removing the bony prominence (5).

Heel Bumps (Haglund's Deformity)

Heel bumps are an enlargement of the bone at the back of the heel, which can encourage bursitis to develop. Various operations are utilized, ranging from bone removal to the "tilting" of bones into a better position to alleviate the problem (5).

Neuroma Surgery

A neuroma is an enlarged nerve, usually between the third and fourth toes caused by nerve irritation and entrapment between bones. The podiatric surgeon routinely removes neuromas under local anesthetic (5). Some podiatric surgeons utilize endoscopic plantar fasciotomy employing minimally invasive techniques to treat this condition.

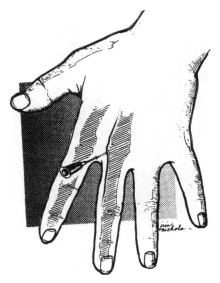

Figure 11.1.   Digital block. Reused with permission from Mulroy MF. (Regional anesthesia: An illustrated procedural guide. 3rd ed. Philadelphia: Lippincott Williams & Wilkins; 2002:196.)

Plantar Fasciitis

An inflammation of the connective tissue found on the underside of the foot. Most patients respond to nonsurgical treatment such as the prescription of orthoses, but on occasion surgery is required. Keyhole techniques are used to treat the condition (5).

Tendon Repair

Any number of foot tendons can be injured causing inflammation and pain and disturbing normal function. A commonly injured tendon is the Achilles tendon. Most patients respond to nonsurgical treatment. On occasion the tendon will be stripped of its inflamed thickened tissue. Tendon lengthening is sometimes required to treat the condition (5).

Anesthetic Technique

Podiatric surgeons will usually administer a local anesthetic, such as lido-caine or bupivacaine, in a local and regional manner, commonly performing *digital or ankle blocks* (see Figures 11.1 and 11.2). When deciding which drug, its dosage, and if any adjuvant medications are going to be used, systemic

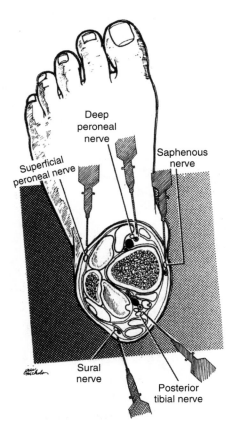

Figure 11.2. Ankle block. Reused with permission from Mulroy MF. (Regional anesthesia: An illustrated procedural guide. 3rd ed. Philadelphia: Lippincott Williams & Wilkins; 2002:222.)

toxicity should be of concern. Often, the local or regional anesthetic will be used in conjunction with an MAC or GA. With GA, whether a LMA or ETT will be used to secure the airway (Table 11.2) will depend on the patient's medical condition and the position of the patient in relation to the anesthesia personnel.

Complications

As with other orthopaedic-type procedures, complications include infection (cellulitis, osteomyelitis), synovitis, tenosynovitis, bone nonunion, and joint contractures.

CARDIAC AND PULMONARY DIAGNOSTIC AND THERAPEUTIC INTERVENTIONS

Depending on the ASA physical status of the patient and the acuity of the condition, the following procedures may be accomplished in the office setting, but often these procedures are performed in the hospital (see Box 11.7).

Box 11.7 • Cardiac and Pulmonary Diagnostic and Therapeutic Interventions

1. Transesophageal Echocardiography
2. Electrocardioversion
3. Bronchoscopy

Transesophageal Echocardiography

A transesophageal echocardiogram (TEE), is an ultrasound that provides an improved view of the heart as seen from an endoscope which is passed through the esophagus. It is typically used to diagnose heart disease and helps determine heart structure, size, and strength, to detect any abnormalities, and to assess the global function.

Electrocardioversion

Patients with non–life-threatening cardiac dysrhythmias, such as atrial fibrillation, who have stable vital signs can undergo electrocardioversion in an attempt to revert them to a sinus rhythm. This can be accomplished in the office, but is typically performed in an outpatient cardiology clinic located within a hospital due to the possibility of these patients becoming unstable.

Bronchoscopy

A bronchoscopy is a diagnostic procedure that provides a view of the tracheobronchial tree (bronchi). These procedures include flexible and rigid bronchoscopy as well as the new Super Dimension (Super D) bronchoscopy. In the latter, an electromagnetic field is created around the subject's chest allowing for three-dimensional analysis and for bronchoscopy instruments to obtain a tissue sample (14). This procedure is typically performed to investigate abnormal chest x-rays, or to collect biopsy bronchial or lung secretions, or to help diagnose and evaluate upper respiratory issues.

Depending on the particular patient, these procedures may require the entire range from a simple sedation to TIVA or GA (Table 11.2). To ensure patient safety, regardless of where the procedure is performed, if any anesthesia is utilized we recommend strict adherence to ASA standards for the anesthetic preparation, patient monitoring, and technique (see Chapter 5).

REFERENCES

1. American Society of Anesthesiologists, Committee on Communications and the Committee on Ambulatory Surgical Care. *Guidelines for office-based anesthesia*. Approved October 1999 and reaffirmed October 2004.
2. Sa Rego MM, Mehernoor FW, White PF. The changing role of monitored anesthesia care in the ambulatory setting. *Anesth Anal*. 1997;85:1020–1036.
3. Coleman WP, Glogau RG, Klein JA, et al. Guidelines of care for liposuction. *J Am Acad Dermatol*. 2001;45:438–447.
4. Iverson RE, Lynch DJ. Practice advisory on liposuction. *Plast Reconstr Surg*. 2004;113(5):1478–1490.
5. Iverson RE. Patient Safety in office based surgical facilities: I. Procedures in the office- based setting. *Plast Reconstr Surg*. 2002;110:1337–1313; discussion 1343–1346.
6. Jaffe RA, Samuels SI. *Anesthesiologist's manual of surgical procedures*, 3rd ed. Philadelphia: Lippincott Williams & Wilkins; 2004:114–137, 892–894, B1–B4.
7. Taghinia AH, Shapiro FE, Slavin SA. Dexmedetomidine in facial aesthetic surgery: Improving anesthetic safety and efficacy. *Plast Reconstr Surg*. In press.
8. Rao RB, Ely SF, Hoffman RS. Deaths related to liposuction. *N Engl J Med*. 1999;340:1471–1475.
9. Sabiston DC Jr. *Textbook of surgery: the biological basis of modern surgical practice*, 5th ed. Philadelphia: WB Saunders; 1997:1327.
10. The Academy of General Dentistry (website). 2005. www.agd.org.
11. The Canadian Dental Association (website). 2005. www.cda-adc.ca.
12. The University of Maryland Medical Center. *Online resources*. 2004. www.umm.edu.
13. Dockery GL, Crawford ME. The Maxwell-brancheau arthroereisis (MBA) implant in pediatric and adult flexible flatfoot conditions. *Foot Ankle Q*. 1999;12(4):107–120.
14. Morgan GE Jr, Mikhail MS, Murray MJ. *Clinical anesthesiology*, 3rd ed. New York: McGraw-Hill; 2002:761–770.
15. Schwartz SI, Shires GT, Spencer FC, et al. *Principles of surgery*, 7th ed. New York: McGraw-Hill; 1999:1337.
16. Barash PG, Cullen BF, Stoelting RK. *Clinical anesthesia*, 4th ed. Philadelphia: Lippincott Williams & Wilkins; 2001:969–988.
17. Southern Ocean County Hospital (website). 2005. www.soch.com.
18. Gildea TR, Mazzone PJ, Karnak D, et al. Electromagnetic navigation diagnostic bronchoscopy: A prospective study. *Am J Respir Crit Care Med*. 2006;174:982–989.
19. Chung F. European Society of Anaesthesiologists. *Refresher courses. Office-based anesthesia: can it be done safely?* April 6, 2002.
20. The Society of Chiropodists and Podiatrists (website). 2005. www.feetforlife.org.

Ophthalmology in the Office

M. Jacob Kaczmarski

In 2005, approximately 2.5 million of the 10 million office-based procedures performed in the United States were ophthalmologic. Cataract surgery is one of the most commonly performed operations yearly in the United States.

Practices may differ considerably amongst physicians for specific types of ophthalmic surgeries. A variety of options for regional and intravenous anesthetics are currently available. Patients presenting for eye surgery range from pediatric to the very elderly, healthy to those with multiple medical comorbidities. An understanding of the anesthetic considerations for ocular procedures is essential to providing safe and efficient outpatient care. To ensure patient safety, regardless of where the procedure is performed, if any anesthesia is utilized we recommend strict adherence to American Society of Anesthesiologists (ASA) standards for the anesthetic preparation, patient monitoring, and technique.

GENERAL CONSIDERATIONS IN OPHTHALMIC ANESTHESIA

Although the vast majority of eye operations and anesthetics are relatively straightforward, the anesthesiologist must exercise careful judgment as to which patients are appropriate candidates for procedures in the office setting.

Sedation and anxiolysis of varying depth in conjunction with a regional anesthetic, such as a retrobulbar block or facial nerve block usually administered by the ophthalmologist, is the typical anesthetic technique utilized. As with any office-based procedure, the use of general anesthesia may be needed and is based on any number of patients or surgical considerations.

Intraocular surgery with regional anesthesia/monitored anesthesia care (MAC) requires significant patient cooperation; movement during the procedure or performance of the block may result in severe complications such as blindness, perforation of the globe, and retrobulbar hemorrhage.

Therefore, patients with conditions such as chronic cough, orthopnea, excessive anxiety, language barrier, or agitation may be better managed with general anesthesia in a hospital or ambulatory surgical center (see Box 12.1).

Box 12.1 • Relative Contraindications to Regional Anesthesia/MAC in Ophthalmology

- Agitation
- Tremor
- Inability to cooperate
- Chronic cough
- Language barrier
- Cognitive impairment
- Orthopnea
- Excessive anxiety

As previously noted, office ophthalmic cases are currently being performed most frequently using a local/regional anesthetic with or without MAC. Typically, patients are treated with a mild sedative, anxiolytic, or short-acting narcotic medication. This can be administered throughout the procedure, or just before performance of the regional technique, which is often the part with the most patient stimulation.

Propofol, remifentanil, and midazolam are intravenous medications that are frequently used individually or in combination during ophthalmic surgery. A one-time propofol bolus before the regional technique has been shown to be safe and effective in reducing patient recall (1), and propofol may continued to be administered throughout the procedure through infusion or bolus dosing without substantial lingering sedation. Remifentanil is popular with outpatient ophthalmologic procedures because it is an ultra short-acting potent analgesic whose effects cease rapidly upon discontinuation. Propofol and remifentanil have been used together with excellent results (2). Midazolam is notable for its anxiolytic and amnestic properties, along with a relatively short half-life. Dexmedetomidine, an α_2 receptor agonist, has been used more recently in the outpatient setting; its benefits stem from its cardiorespiratory sparing effects and its ability to decrease the requirements of other sedatives. An important point to remember is that patient sedation should be titrated to a level at which the patient is alert enough to cooperate with the requests of the ophthalmologist.

Standard monitoring (see Chapter 5) provides adequate surveillance during ophthalmic surgeries. The head of the table is usually rotated 90 or 180 degrees away from the anesthesiologist. Supplemental oxygen should be administered throughout the procedure, preferably with end-tidal CO_2 monitoring. A nasal cannula is sufficient in most cases and will not intrude onto the surgical field. The intravenous line should be placed so that it is easily accessible throughout the case, and efforts should be made to keep a direct line of vision in order to observe the patient's face. Drapes should be organized in a manner that maximizes patient comfort.

REGIONAL ANESTHESIA

The three major regional techniques performed in ophthalmology procedures are retrobulbar, peribulbar, and sub-Tenon's nerve blocks (see Table 12.1). All are widely used and accepted in clinical practice, and the first two may be performed by both anesthesiologists and ophthalmologists. The terms *retrobulbar* and *peribulbar* are used to differentiate whether the injection of local anesthetic is made inside or outside of the cone formed by the extraocular muscles. Tenon's capsule is a semiopaque fibrous tissue layer in which local anesthetic solution can be injected. It is found underneath the conjunctiva and inserts circumferentially 1 mm posterior to the limbus. A small surgical dissection is required to access this space. Regional techniques can provide the necessary anesthesia, akinesia, and hypotonia required for eye surgery when performed properly. These conditions are especially important with more intricate ocular surgeries. Many factors play a role in determining

Table 12.1. A comparison of regional techniques in ophthalmic surgery

Retrobulbar Block	Peribulbar Block	Sub-Tenon's Block
Needle insertion	Needle insertion	Blunt probe/cannula
Rapid onset	Slower onset	Rapid onset
One or two injections	Up to four injections	Single surgical dissection
Smaller volume	Larger volume	Smaller volume
Inside muscle cone	Outside muscle cone	Sub-Tenon's space
Higher risk	Lower risk	Lower risk

the safety and efficacy of regional anesthesia in ophthalmologic surgery. These include the experience of the physician, knowledge of orbital anatomy and physiology, composition of the anesthetic solution, patient positioning, and the type of equipment used.

Researchers at the Johns Hopkins University performed a literature review and data analysis to compare the effectiveness of regional techniques for cataract surgery (3). Two of the conclusions from the study were that peribulbar and retrobulbar blocks provide equivalent akinesia and intra-operative pain control. However, there still exists much variation in the choice of regional technique in most clinical situations and opinions about efficacy.

Peribulbar Anesthesia

Peribulbar injection of local anesthetic outside of the muscle cone may be considered a safer and equally effective alternative to retrobulbar injections (4) because there remains a greater distance between the needle tip and the globe. Because of the location of the injection, the block requires a greater amount of local anesthetic (6–8 mL) and a longer time to effect. Also, orbital compression should be applied after the injections to minimize an increase in intraocular pressure and to facilitate local anesthetic spread. The injectate usually takes several minutes to reach the insertion sites of the oculomotor nerves into the extraocular muscles by diffusion.

Peribulbar regional anesthesia has been customarily performed using a series of up to four injections, but recently, a single injection technique obtained satisfactory and equivalent results (5). Common approaches involve two injections using a blunt tipped, 25- to 27-gauge needle approximately $1\frac{1}{4}$ in. long. The injections are placed inferotemporally and superonasally just beyond the equator of the globe. The needle should not be advanced a distance >25 mm, and always aspirated before injection to rule out accidental intravascular location.

Some practitioners initially perform one of the injections, observe the efficacy, and then decide to perform a second at a different site if necessary. Therefore, variations of the traditional peribulbar injection technique are frequently utilized depending on operator experience and preference.

Retrobulbar Anesthesia

The retrobulbar injection of local anesthetic has historically been the most popular manner of delivering anesthetic behind and around the globe. Retrobulbar blockade is viewed as producing more reliable anesthesia and akinesia with a smaller volume of anesthetic ($\sim$4 mL), albeit with a higher risk of complications. The retrobulbar block is performed using a sharp, small gauge needle (25–27 gauge), using a single injection technique. The needle is often slightly longer than those used for peribulbar blockade. The injection is made in the infratemporal quadrant, again with careful aspiration for blood or cerebrospinal fluid (CSF). Retrobulbar blocks do not provide akinesia of the accompanying eyelid, and a separate injection is therefore utilized to achieve blockade of the facial nerve.

Sub-Tenon's Block

Sub-Tenon's block has emerged as a fairly recent alternative to retrobulbar and peribulbar injections, as well as topical anesthesia, in ophthalmologic surgery. A study in the British Journal of Ophthalmology concluded that it is a safe and effective alternative to peribulbar blocks in both anterior and posterior segment eye surgery (6) and data also suggests that sub-Tenon's block is superior to topical anesthesia for cataract surgery with a similar amount of complications (7). The sub-Tenon's block is unique in that a small dissection into the conjunctiva is performed before the injection of anesthetic

Table 12.2.   Regional anesthetic solutions in ophthalmology

Short acting: Lidocaine 2%	Long acting: Bupivacaine 0.5% or 0.75%
Epinephrine 1/400,000	Hyaluronidase 3 U/mL

through a blunt tipped cannula. The rationale for the procedure comes from the fact that an anesthetic solution injected into the posterior aspect of sub-Tenon's space will reach the contents of the retrobulbar area through diffusion. The volume of injectate and onset to action are similar to that of retrobulbar blockade.

PATIENT POSITION

The classic "Atkinson" positioning of the eye before the regional technique has been replaced by the more recent "primary gaze" position. In the former, the patient was instructed to look in a superomedial direction. This has been shown to displace the optic nerve in a manner that places it in closer proximity to the path of the retrobulbar needle. Patients are now instructed to look directly ahead during performance of the block (8,9).

It is critical to ensure that the patient has an appropriate head position before beginning surgery. Typically, the infraorbital and supraorbital rims should be parallel to the floor. In this way, the surgeon is able to rotate the globe an equal distance superiorly as well as inferiorly during surgery. In addition, in patients with deep set eyes, the surgeon is best able to access the globe without working over the steep brow.

ANESTHETIC SOLUTION

The constituents of the retrobulbar and peribulbar blocks typically include a short- and long-acting anesthetic (see Table 12.2). A 50/50 mixture of 2% lidocaine with 0.75% bupivacaine is commonly used. Epinephrine (1:400,000 dilution) is often added to the mixture to decrease bleeding and prolong the local anesthetic effects. Finally, hyaluronidase, which catalyzes the hydrolysis of hyaluronic acid and therefore increases tissue permeability, is sometimes added to help facilitate orbital infiltration of the medication.

COMPLICATIONS OF REGIONAL ANESTHESIA

Retrobulbar hemorrhage is a potentially serious complication of peribulbar and retrobulbar injections (see Box 12.2). The origin of the bleeding may be either arterial or venous. Arterial bleeding is characterized by a more rapid rise in intraocular pressure and prominent proptosis. Such an increase in intraocular pressure is dangerous because retinal perfusion may be compromised by compression of the retinal artery. Treatment of retrobulbar hemorrhage includes immediate manual compression of the orbit. Pharmacologic treatments to lower intraocular pressure may be necessary, as is a lateral canthotomy or anterior chamber paracentesis in the most serious cases (10). The scheduled surgical procedure should be cancelled. Superficial hemorrhage and hematoma formation are other less serious bleeding-related complications. An important point to realize is that a significant number of patients presenting for ophthalmologic procedures will be taking some sort of oral anticoagulant. A prospective study examining approximately 20,000 cataract surgeries performed on patients taking oral anticoagulants and /or antiplatelet medications found that the rates of medical or surgical complications were extremely low, and absolute differences as to the risk/benefit ratio of continuing or discontinuing these medications could not be established (11).

Box 12.2 • Various Complications of Regional Anesthesia in Ophthalmology

- Retrobulbar hemorrhage
- Brainstem anesthesia
- Extraocular muscle damage
- Globe perforation
- Local anesthetic toxicity
- Hematoma formation
- Oculocardiac reflex (OCR)
- Optic nerve damage

Another potential complication of regional anesthesia is *penetration or perforation of the globe*. The globe may be penetrated by the needle either one or two times; at the entry and exit points respectively. Several factors have been determined that place patients at an increased risk for this complication. These include an axial diameter >26 mm, a patient who requires multiple injections to achieve satisfactory anesthesia, or an uncooperative patient. Some physicians feel that the presence of a scleral buckle also increases risk. Most globe perforation injuries will resolve without intervention; however, vitrectomy is occasionally indicated. Direct trauma to the optic nerve is a rare but deadly complication that in severe cases may result in permanent vision loss.

The *oculocardiac reflex (OCR)* is a vagal response mediated through the trigeminal nerve that principally manifests itself as bradycardia and hypotension (see Box 12.3). It may be elicited by manipulation and stimulation of the eyeball, such as what occurs during the performance of a nerve block or surgical maneuvers. It is most commonly seen during strabismus surgery in pediatric patients. The symptoms usually resolve upon discontinuation of the stimulus. Atropine may be used if the bradycardia persists. Electrocardiogram (EKG) monitoring during all ophthalmologic procedures is of utmost importance.

Box 12.3 • The Oculocardiac Reflex

- Owing to external pressure or traction on the extraocular muscles eliciting a trigeminovagal reflex arc
- May manifest as somnolence (awake patients), bradycardia, ventricular ectopy, sinus arrest, and ventricular fibrillation; electrocardiographic monitoring essential
- Prevented by retrobulbar block, anticholinergics, deepening anesthesia
- Treatment involves ceasing causative stimulus, assessing depth of anesthesia, and atropine for bradycardia

---

Preoperative use of intravenous anticholinergic medications, such as atropine or glycopyrrolate, approximately 30 minutes before surgery, is often helpful in preventing this reflex; intramuscular premedication is not as efficacious (see Box 12.4) (12,13).

Box 12.4 • Management of the Oculocardiac Reflex

1. Immediate notification of the surgeon and temporary cessation of surgical stimulation
2. Confirmation of adequate ventilation, oxygenation, and anesthetic depth
3. Administration of atropine (10 μg/kg IV) if the condition persists
4. Infiltration of local anesthetic during recalcitrant episodes

---

Brainstem anesthesia is a result of the entrance of local anesthetic to the central nervous system (CNS) through the optic nerve sheath, and may present as the gradual development of contralateral amaurosis and deterioration of pulmonary, cardiovascular, and neurologic functioning. Accidental intra-arterial injection of the contents of a regional block is heralded by the immediate development of seizures. Equipment and drugs necessary for advanced cardiopulmonary resuscitation should therefore always be readily available.

Postoperative diplopia, strabismus, or *ptosis* may be a sign of extraocular muscle damage. Etiologies include trauma, local anesthetic–induced myotoxicity, or pressure damage from surgical devices or the volume of injected medication.

EYE MEDICATION AND SYSTEMIC EFFECTS

Locally administered ophthalmic medications can be readily absorbed into the systemic circulation (see Box 12.5). Although administered topically in small amounts, they are highly concentrated and may have notable systemic effects.

Box 12.5

Common Medications in Ophthalmologic Surgery

Phenylephrine	Cyclopentolate
Echothiophate	Acetazolamide
Timolol/Betaxolol	Epinephrine

Phenylephrine is used to create mydriasis and vasoconstriction during surgery. Absorption may cause headache, arrhythmias, and severe hypertension, which may precipitate myocardial ischemia.

Echothiophate is an irreversible cholinesterase inhibitor used in treating glaucoma. Its systemic absorption may lead to a reduction in plasma pseudocholinesterase activity for up to 4 to 6 weeks after its discontinuation. Prolonged paralysis and apnea, when given the usual dose of succinylcholine, is a risk and should be anticipated. Paralysis usually does not exceed 20 to 30 minutes.

Timolol is a nonselective β-blocker used to decrease production of aqueous humor. It may cause bradycardia, congestive heart failure (CHF), hypotension, and exacerbate asthma. Betaxolol is a newer β_1 selective agent that may have less potential to produce systemic effects.

Cyclopentolate drops are used to cause mydriasis. Confusion, dysarthria, and seizures due to CNS toxicity are possible.

Acetazolamide is a carbonic anhydrase inhibitor and diuretic. It is used to decrease intraocular pressure and may cause a hypokalemic metabolic acidosis.

Epinephrine may cause hypertension, tachycardia, and arrhythmias.

OPHTHALMOLOGIC SURGERIES
Procedures

Ophthalmologic surgeries can be broadly categorized as either intraocular or extraocular surgery. The two most common forms of extraocular surgery include strabismus surgery and retinal detachment surgery; however, the latter can involve intraocular involvement if the surgeon elects to perforate and drain the subretinal fluid. The following is a brief list of intraocular, or open-eye, surgical procedures (see Box 12.6) (13,14).

Box 12.6 • Commonly Performed Ophthalmologic Procedures

1. Cataract extraction
2. Corneal laceration
3. Removal of foreign body
4. Retinal surgery
5. Ruptured globe repair
6. Trabeculectomy
7. Vitrectomy

Cataract Extraction

Cataract extraction is the leading cause of treatable blindness in the world and is defined as opacification of the crystalline lens. Cataract removal is an extremely common procedure associated with excellent results. Modern cataract surgery is performed using the extracapsular technique, or removal of the cataract contents through an anterior lens capsulectomy and corneal incision. Phacoemulsification, or ultrasound fragmentation of the cataract nucleus, only requires a corneal incision of approximately 3 mm through which the contents are aspirated. A synthetic intraocular lens, often silicon or acrylic, is then implanted through the same opening. The incision may then be closed with sutures; however, it is frequently self-sealing. Blood loss, pain, and operative time are minimal. Topical antibiotics are frequently administered by the surgeon. Routine preoperative medical testing for cataract removal has not been shown to increase patient safety (15).

Corneal Laceration Repair

Laceration of the cornea may heal spontaneously or, depending on depth, may require primary closure.

Corneal Transplant (Penetrating Keratoplasty)

Corneal transplant, or penetrating keratoplasty, is used to replace scarred, swollen, or otherwise damaged corneas resulting in visual impairment. The patient's cornea is replaced with tissue from a donor. A small piece is removed from the patient's cornea using a trephine, and a slightly larger piece of tissue from the donor is then sutured into position. Operative time is usually approximately 1 hour.

Removal of Foreign Body

See discussion on *ruptured globe repair* in the subsequent text.

Retinal Surgery

Retinal surgery usually involves the repair of a retinal tear or detachment resulting from a number of conditions including trauma, postcataract extraction, and diabetic retinopathy, amongst others. It can also involve the surgical correction of macular disease. A number of different procedures can be employed to achieve the desired results. Although most of these procedures can be performed in the outpatient office setting under local anesthesia or MAC, depending on the length of the procedure (<2 hours), general anesthesia may be used. Hospitalization may be required depending on the cause of the eye condition and any patient comorbidities.

Ruptured Globe Repair

This condition involves the tear of either the cornea or sclera typically resulting from a traumatic injury. Surgical repair involves replacing intraocular contents, closing defects, and removing foreign objects. This procedure is typically performed under general anesthesia.

Trabeculectomy and Other Filtering Procedures

Trabeculectomy is the most common surgical procedure to treat glaucoma and reduce intraocular pressure. Glaucoma, or optic nerve damage due to elevated intraocular pressure, is second only to cataract as the leading cause of blindness worldwide. Trabeculectomy involves the creation of a passageway between the anterior chamber and subconjunctival space, allowing drainage of aqueous humor and relief of the excess pressure. The most common complication of trabeculectomy involves the proliferation of scar tissue and disruption of the filtration channel. Mitomycin-C or 5-fluorouracil may be applied topically by the surgeon in the hope of preventing fibroblast proliferation.

Vitrectomy (Anterior and Posterior)

Vitrectomy, the removal of vitreous humor from the eye, is a surgical procedure involved in treating several types of ocular pathology such as proliferative diabetic retinopathy, retinal detachment, foreign body removal, and endophthalmitis. The vitreous gel is removed using microsurgical instruments to obtain access to the posterior portion of the eye and retina. Once access is obtained, numerous other procedures may occur. Membranectomy removes unhealthy tissue layers from the retina. Laser photocoagulation is used to seal retinal holes and shrink blood vessels. A scleral buckle may be added as a supportive structure to ensure the retina remains properly in place. Intraocular gases (perfluoropropane, C_3F_8 and sulfur hexafluoride, SF_6) or silicone oil is also frequently used to serve as a substitute for the removed vitreous gel and aid in securing the retina after surgery. A patient must be able to tolerate a "face down" position for 2 to 3 weeks postoperatively after injection of an intraocular gas. The patient will also experience distorted vision until the majority of the gas is replaced by new ocular fluid.

Patients who receive silicone oil are not required to maintain certain positions and are able to see normally. However, the silicone is not reabsorbed by the body and another surgery may be required to remove it from the eye.

Complications

Postoperative ocular complications include corneal abrasion (most commonly), chemical injury, photic injury (resulting from laser use), mild visual disturbances (i.e., photophobia and diplopia), hemorrhagic retinopathy, retinal ischemia, and ischemic optic neuropathy.

CONCLUSION

The trend toward the performance of more ophthalmologic procedures in the office setting is likely to continue to grow. Educated and well-informed anesthesiology personnel are the key to maintaining both the success of this increase along with patient safety.

REFERENCES

 1. Habib NE, Balmer HG, Hocking G. Efficacy and safety of sedation with propofol in peribulbar anaesthesia. *Eye.* 2002;16(1):60–62.
 2. Rewari V, Madan R, Kaul HL, et al. Remifentanil and propofol sedation for retrobulbar nerve block. *Anaesth Intensive Care.* 2002;30(4):433–437.
 3. Friedman DS, Bass EB, Lubomski LH. Synthesis of the literature on the effectiveness of regional anesthesia for cataract surgery. *Ophthalmology.* 2001;108(3):519–529.
 4. Davis DB II, Mandel MR. Efficacy and complication rate of 16,224 consecutive peribulbar blocks. A prospective multicenter study. *J Cataract Refract Surg.* 1994;20(3):327–337.
 5. Rizzo L, Marini M, Rosati C, et al. Peribulbar anesthesia: A percutaneous single injection technique with a small volume of anesthetic. *Anesth Analg.* 2005;100(1):94–96.
 6. Roman SJ, Chong Sit DA, Boureau CM, et al. Sub-Tenon's anaesthesia: An efficient and safe technique. *Br J Ophthalmol.* 1997;81(8):673–676.
 7. Srinivasan S, Fern AI, Selvaraj S, et al. Randomized double-blind clinical trial comparing topical and sub-Tenon's anaesthesia in routine cataract surgery. *Br J Anaesth.* 2004;93(5):683–686.
 8. Liu C, Youl B, Moseley I. Magnetic resonance imaging of the optic nerve in extremes of gaze. Implications for the positioning of the globe for retrobulbar anaesthesia. *Br J Ophthalmol.* 1992;76(12):728–733.
 9. Unsold R, Stanley JA, DeGroot J. The CT-topography of retrobulbar anesthesia. Anatomic-clinical correlation of complications and suggestion of a modified technique. *Albrecht Von Graefes Arch Klin Exp Ophthalmol.* 1981;217(2):125–136.
10. Duker JS, Belmont JB, Benson WE, et al. Inadvertent globe perforation during retrobulbar and peribulbar anesthesia. Patient characteristics, surgical management, and visual outcome. *Ophthalmology.* 1991;98(4):519–526.
11. Katz J, Feldman MA, Bass EB, et al. Study of Medical Testing for Cataract Surgery Team. Risks and benefits of anticoagulant and antiplatelet medication use before cataract surgery. *Ophthalmology.* 2003;110(9):1784–1788; Erratum in: *Ophthalmology.* 2003;110(12):2309.
12. Schwartz SI, Shires GT, Spencer FC, et al. *Principles of surgery,* 7th ed. New York: McGraw-Hill; 1999:1337.
13. Barash PG, Cullen BF, Stoelting RK. *Clinical anesthesia,* 4th ed. Philadelphia: Lippincott Williams & Wilkins; 2001:969–988.
14. Iverson RE. Patient safety in office based surgical facilities: I. Procedures in the office-based setting. *Plast Reconstr Surg.* 2002;110:1337–1342; discussion 1343–1346.
15. Schein OD, Katz J, Bass EB, et al. Study of Medical Testing for Cataract Surgery Study Team. The value of routine preoperative medical testing before cataract surgery. *N Engl J Med.* 2000;342:168–175.

Gastrointestinal Endoscopy in the Office-Based Setting

Kai Matthes

Endoscopic procedures are typically performed in an office or ambulatory surgical center and rarely in a hospital operating room. A total of 2.8 million sigmoidoscopies and 14.2 million colonoscopies were performed in the United States in 2002 (1). This number has continued to rise exponentially along with the increased number of diagnostic and interventional procedures being performed.

An integral part of the practice of gastrointestinal (GI) endoscopy is adequate sedation and analgesia. The level of sedation required depends on the type of endoscopic procedure being performed. Most endoscopies are performed with patients under "conscious sedation." At this level of consciousness, the patient is able to make a purposeful response to verbal or tactile stimulation, and both ventilatory and cardiovascular function are maintained. There are instances that require a greater depth of sedation that can lead to general anesthesia.

To clarify this point, the American Society of Anesthesiologists (ASA) has classified four "levels" of sedation (see Table 13.1). By comparison, patient responsiveness during "deep sedation" involves purposeful responses to painful stimuli only. Airway support is sometimes required to maintain sufficient oxygenation (2). At the level of general anesthesia, the patient is not arousable, even to painful stimuli. Airway support is frequently required and cardiovascular function may be impaired (2–4).

Sedation for upper GI endoscopy is considered safe, with only minimal risk for the patient. However, cardiopulmonary complications may account for more than 50% of all reported complications. Most of these incidents are based on the following:

- Vasovagal episodes
- Oversedation
- Hypoventilation
- Aspiration
- Airway obstruction (5,6)

A prospective survey of 14,149 upper endoscopies indicated that the rate of immediate cardiopulmonary incidents was 2 per 1,000 cases with a 30-day mortality rate of 1 per 2,000 cases (7). A retrospective review of 21,011 procedures found the rate of cardiovascular complications was 5.4 per 1,000 procedures (8). The reported complications varied from mild transient hypoxemia to severe cardiorespiratory compromise and death.

To ensure patient safety, regardless of where the procedure is performed, if any anesthesia is utilized strict adherence to ASA standards for the anesthetic preparation, patient monitoring, and technique is recommended (see Chapter 5). In addition to the details mentioned in the preceding text, the American Gastroenterological Association (AGA) also established a standard

Table 13.1.   Continuum of depth of sedation—definition of general anesthesia and levels of sedation/analgesia[a]

	Minimal Sedation (Anxiolysis)	Moderate Sedation/Analgesia (Conscious Sedation)	Deep Sedation/Analgesia	General Anesthesia
Responsiveness	Normal response to verbal stimulation	Purposeful response to verbal or tactile stimulation	Purposeful response following repeated or painful stimulation	Unarousable even with painful stimulus
Airway	Unaffected	No intervention required	Intervention may be required	Intervention often required
Spontaneous ventilation	Unaffected	Adequate	May be inadequate	Frequently inadequate
Cardiovascular function	Unaffected	Usually maintained	Usually maintained	May be impaired

[a]http://www.asahq.org/publicationsAndServices/standards/20.pdf

that an anesthesia risk class should be documented for each patient receiving intravenous sedation, using the ASA score (30). Simply stated:

1. Patients with an ASA score of III should be further assessed for their appropriateness to undergo in-office endoscopy.
2. Patients with an ASA score of IV should not undergo in-office endoscopy.

CHOICE OF ANESTHETIC REGIMEN
Anesthetic Technique

Sedation and anxiolysis have in the past been administered by the endoscopist; however, it has become increasingly more common to have an anesthesiologist present during these procedures.

Sedation for GI endoscopy is particularly challenging because of the variability in long nonstimulating periods with intermitted peak stimulating events. Some endoscopic procedures may be undertaken without sedation. Most of the cases are performed under a monitored anesthesia care (MAC) anesthetic but occasionally general anesthesia is required for patients who are unable to tolerate these procedures under sedation alone.

The following patient characteristics were associated with tolerance of upper endoscopy or colonoscopy, with little or no sedation in a number of clinical trials:

- Elderly
- Anxious patients
- Male gender
- Absence of abdominal pain history

Less well studied are the factors that predict which patients are prone to experience great difficulty with sedation. The characteristics of "difficult to sedate" patients are recognized by most experienced endoscopists (see Box 13.1).

Box 13.1 • Increased Anesthetic Requirement

- A history of prior difficulty with conscious sedation
- Prescribed or illicit benzodiazepine or opiates use
- Heavy alcohol use

Monitored Anesthesia Care

MAC requires intensive monitoring by trained individuals. Related risk factors, the depth of sedation, and the urgency of the endoscopic procedure play important roles in determining whether or not an anesthesiologist is consulted. The choice of medication for deep sedation during endoscopic retrograde cholangiopancreatography (ERCP) is largely operator dependent, but generally consists of sedatives such as propofol or a benzodiazepine used either alone or in combination with an opiate. The most commonly used benzodiazepines are midazolam and diazepam, favoring midazolam because of its fast onset, short duration, and high amnestic properties. Doses are titrated to patient tolerance depending on age, other illnesses, use of additional medications, and the sedation requirements of the particular procedure. For prolonged therapeutic procedures, such as ERCP, propofol

Table 13.2.   Anesthetics

Drug	Bolus Dose (IV)	Infusion Rate (IV)
Diazepam	5–10 mg	
Midazolam	0.5–7.5 mg[a]	1–2 μg/kg/min
Propofol	20–100 mg	25–75 μg/kg/min
Thiopental	50–150 mg	
Methohexital	10–20 mg	20–60 μg/kg/min
Ketamine	20–40 mg	5–20 μg/kg/min
Dexmedetomidine	1 μg/kg over 10 min	0.1–0.7 μg/kg/h

[a] Lower dosage in elderly or in combination with second sedative, higher dosage if used alone without additional sedative

has been demonstrated to be advantageous when compared with standard benzodiazepine/narcotic sedation in terms of faster onset, deeper sedation, and faster recovery (2,9–20). Deep sedation requires intensive monitoring by individuals trained in emergency resuscitation and airway management. (see Chapter 5)

Sedatives/Anxiolytics

Patients undergoing MAC for GI endoscopy may be premedicated with a benzodiazepine, preferably midazolam, due to its rapid onset and short-acting properties. Propofol is preferred over other anesthetics because of its rapid onset and short, time-independent, context-sensitive half-time. Dexmedetomidine is an α_2 agonist with sedative, analgesic, anxiolytic, and MAC-sparing properties, along with hemodynamic and respiratory stability. These characteristics make this drug promising for conscious or deeper levels of sedation. It is currently indicated for the use of sedation in the intensive care unit (ICU) setting for 24 hours. However, in 2007, it is scheduled to undergo phase III clinical trials for an U.S. Food and Drug Administration (FDA)-approved indication for its perioperative use in MAC cases (see Tables 13.2 and 13.3). Table 13.2 includes dexmedetomidine with the recommended dosing.

Most endoscopic procedures do not require strong analgesics as there are usually only limited periods of modest stimulation. Fentanyl may be given in small boluses as an adjunct to the anesthetic regimen. Remifentanil provides a strong analgesic effect and offers the advantage of a time-independent context-sensitive half-life. The ventilatory depressant effects of narcotics should be noted, especially when used in combination with other sedatives. Caution should be exercised in patients undergoing MAC for endoscopy due

Table 13.3.   Analgesics

Drug	Bolus Dose	Infusion Rate
Fentanyl	25–50 μg	
Alfentanil	0.25–0.75 mg	
Remifentanil	12.5–25 μg	0.025–0.15 μg/kg/min
Nalbuphine	5–15 mg	
Ketorolac	15–30 mg	

Table 13.4. Induction

Drug	Induction Dose (IV)
Propofol	2.0–2.5 mg/kg
Thiopental	3–5 mg/kg
Ketamine	1–1.5 mg/kg
Fentanyl	1 μg/kg

to unprotected airway, the potential to become apneic, and the potential for aspiration.

Pharyngeal Anesthesia

Commonly used topical anesthetics include benzocaine, tetracaine, and lidocaine, which are administered by aerosol spray or gargling. Topical benzocaine is effective to prevent the gag reflex during insertion of the endoscope. The application should be limited to a single spray of no more than 1-second duration in order to avoid methemoglobulinemia, a systemic side effect that may result from multiple topical doses. Methemoglobinemia is a condition in which hemoglobin becomes oxidized and converted from the ferrous state (Fe^{2+}) to the ferric state (Fe^{3+} = methemoglobin). Methemoglobin lacks the electron that is needed to form a bond with oxygen, therefore oxygen transport is prevented, which ultimately results in clinical hypoxia.

General Anesthesia

Some patients may require general anesthesia, if sedation alone is insufficient for the patient to tolerate the procedure (see Table 13.4).

Maintenance of General Anesthesia

Maintenance of anesthesia during endoscopy can be achieved with inhalation anesthetics. Rarely, muscle relaxation may be required if patients need to be absolutely motionless during ERCP.

PATIENT MONITORING FOR GASTROINTESTINAL ENDOSCOPY

According to the guidelines of the ASA (see Chapter 5) and American Society for Gastrointestinal Endoscopy (ASGE) for conscious sedation and monitoring during GI endoscopy, patients undergoing endoscopic procedures with moderate or deep sedation must have continuous monitoring before, during, and after the administration of sedatives (see Boxes 13.2 and 13.3) (4).

Box 13.2

Standard Noninvasive Monitoring
- Blood pressure[1]
- Electrocardiogram (ECG)[1]
- Oxygen and gas analyzer
- Pulse oximetry (SaO_2)[1]
- Capnography
- Transcutaneous electrical nerve stimulation
- Body temperature

[1]Minimal monitoring requirement during monitored anesthesia care for gastrointestinal endoscopy

---

Box 13.3

Standard Anesthetic Equipment
- Anesthesia machine
- Oral suction
- Emergency drugs (atropine, phenylephrine, succinylcholine)
- Airway equipment (laryngoscope, endotracheal tubes, Ambu-bag)

Supplemental Oxygen

Supplemental oxygen administration has been shown conclusively in controlled trials to reduce the incidence of desaturation, which can occur in up to 47% of patients undergoing ERCP without oxygen (21,22). However, supplemental oxygen may mask hypoventilation (23,24). Pulse oximetry is a "late sign" of airway obstruction; hypercarbia occurs *before* hypoxia becomes evident with a decrease of SaO_2 values. During hypoventilation, a significant amount of CO_2 can accumulate in the patient, which may lead to CO_2 narcosis, before hypoxia becomes evident in desaturation. Therefore, capnography is a more reliable monitor of ventilation.

Capnography

Particularly in prolonged therapeutic procedures such as ERCP, in which deeper levels of sedation are reached, capnography (end-tidal CO_2 monitoring) may be superior for evaluation of ventilation compared with pulse oximetry alone (see Figure 13.1) (25,26). However, routine measurement of CO_2 has not yet been associated with any objective clinical outcome benefits. Oxygen insufflation using nasal prongs combined with an extra nasal capnography line are currently available (see Figure 13.2). Alternatively one can

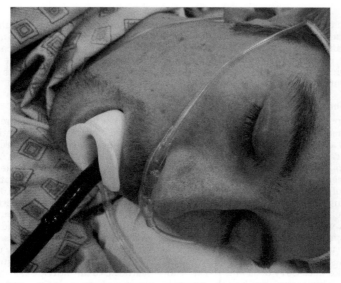

Figure 13.1. Capnography monitoring method A—setup of the Salter CO_2 monitoring nasal cannula. The cannula contains two lumens, one to insufflate oxygen to the patient, and the second is the CO_2 aspiration line.

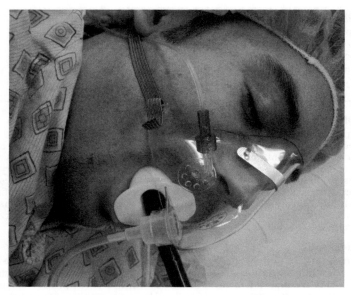

Figure 13.2. Capnography monitoring method B—setup of a standard oxygen face mask adjusted by the lower part of the mask being removed with scissors to facilitate the introduction of the endoscope into the patient's mouth. A regular capnography line is connected to a plastic Luer Lock needle, which is fixed into the side opening of the face mask to detect exhaled CO_2.

attach a plastic syringe needle to a standard capnography line. This can then be fixed into the side holes of the oxygen face mask near the mouth in close proximity to the exhaled air stream (see Figure 13.3). Percutaneous capnography devices are becoming increasingly available and may provide more reliable data than end-tidal CO_2 detection techniques during spontaneous ventilation.

Bispectral Index Monitoring

Bispectral index (BIS) monitoring augments the assessment of the level of consciousness and can act as an adjuvant in determining the etiology of intraoperative events such as hypotension, hypertension, tachycardia, or bradycardia. Using a sensor placed on the patient's forehead, BIS (Aspect Medical Systems Inc., Newton, MA) translates information from the electroencephalogram (EEG) into a single number that represents each patient's level of consciousness. This number—the BIS value—ranges from 100 (indicating an awake patient) to zero (indicating the absence of brain activity). Although there are currently no standardized recommendations about BIS target values for GI endoscopy, a BIS range of 70 to 80 may correspond to an appropriate level of sedation for GI endoscopy with an Observer's Assessment of Alertness/Sedation (OAA/S) score of 3 (see subsequent text) (27). By utilizing this BIS value as a guide intraoperatively, clinicians are better equipped to make necessary decisions to tailor an anesthetic to an individual's specific needs. This technology has the potential to prevent oversedation or intraoperative awareness. It is commercially available; however, it is not currently used as a standard monitoring device for routine endoscopy (28).

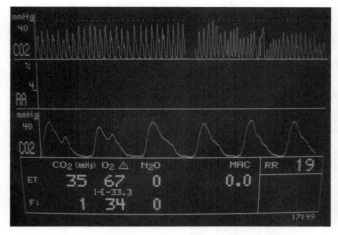

Figure 13.3.   Capnography tracing of monitoring methods A and B.

ASSESSMENT OF SEDATION

An assessment of vigilance can be undertaken using an OAA/S scale (see Table 13.5) (29).

COMMON PROCEDURES IN GASTROINTESTINAL ENDOSCOPY
Esophagogastroduodenoscopy

Esophagogastroduodenoscopy (EGD) is the diagnostic and/or therapeutic examination of the upper GI tract using a flexible endoscope (see Box 13.4). It provides a view from the mouth to the beginning of the small bowel. This procedure is typically performed on patients who have difficulty swallowing or who may have ulcers, heartburn, upper GI bleeding, or to find the cause of abdominal pain. It is also used to investigate tumors or abnormalities in the upper GI tract, and obtain tissue specimens by performing a mucosal biopsy or staining of GI layers. Diagnostic EGD can be performed with little or no sedation, but potentially painful procedures such as, for example, esophageal dilatation require adequate anesthesia.

Box 13.4

Stimulating Events during Esophagogastroduodenoscopy
1. Intubation of the esophagus
2. Passing the scope through the pylorus
3. Endoscopic intervention:
   a. Esophageal/gastric/duodenal biopsy
   b. Endoscopic mucosal resection (EMR)
   c. Endoscopic submucosal dissection (ESD)
   d. Argon plasma coagulation (APC)
   e. Endoscopic hemostasis
   f. Dilatation of esophageal strictures
   g. Esophageal stenting
   h. Photodynamic therapy

Table 13.5. Observer's Assessment and Alertness/Sedation (OAA/S) Scale

OAA/S Score	Patient Response	Speech	Facial Expression	Eyes
5	Responds readily to name spoken in normal tone	Normal	Normal	Clear, no ptosis
4	Lethargic response to name spoken in normal tone	Mild slowing or thickening	Mild relaxation	Glazed or mild ptosis (less than half the eye)
3	Responds only after name is called loudly and/or repeatedly	Slurring or prominent slowing	Marked relaxation	Glazed and marked ptosis (more than half the eye)
2	Responds only after mild prodding or shaking	Few recognizable words		
1	Responds only after squeezing the trapezius			
0	Does not respond after squeezing the trapezius			

From: Chernik DA, Gillings D, Laine H, et al. Validity and reliability of the observer's assessment of alertness/sedation scale: Study with intravenous midazolam. *J Clin Psychopharmacol.* 1990;10:244–251.

Proctoscopy/Sigmoidoscopy/Colonoscopy

Procedures

Proctoscopy is the examination of the rectum using a rigid endoscope, which usually does not require intravenous anesthesia. Sigmoidoscopy is the diagnostic and/or interventional examination of the sigmoid. A colonoscopy provides a view of the interior lining of the large intestine (colon) using a colonoscope, a flexible fiber-optic tube. The procedure provides a view of the entire lower GI tract, extending from the large bowel to the distal ileum. A biopsy may be performed to evaluate tissue, such as hemorrhoids, rectal bleeding, and polyps, or in determining the extent of inflammatory bowel disease. A colonoscopy also helps diagnose colon cancer (see Box 13.5).

Box 13.5

Stimulating Events during Proctoscopy/Sigmoidoscopy/Colonoscopy
1. Introduction of the endoscope
2. Advancement of the endoscope against the bowel wall (diverticula, flexures etc.)
3. Looping of the colonoscope with consecutive distention of the bowel
4. Endoscopic intervention:
   a. Mucosal biopsy
   b. Endoscopic mucosal resection (EMR)
   c. Argon plasma coagulation (APC)
   d. Endoscopic hemostasis
   e. Polypectomy
   f. Dilatation and stenting of malignant strictures

Endoscopic Retrograde Cholangiopancreatography

The ERCP examines the pancreatic and gall bladder ducts and biliary ducts. It can identify and remove stones or tumors in the ducts or identify a narrowing of the ducts.

ERCP is a radiographic examination whereby contrast dye is injected endoscopically through the major or minor duodenal papilla. This procedure requires the skillful delivery of sedation and analgesia. If the patients are too lightly sedated, they move, retch, or gag. If they are too deeply sedated, they may develop airway obstruction, hypoventilation, hemodynamic instability, and delayed emergence and recovery (see Box 13.6).

Box 13.6

Stimulating Events during Endoscopic Retrograde Cholangiopancreatography
1. Intubation of the esophagus
2. Passing the scope through the pylorus
3. Shortening the scope
4. Cannulating the common bile duct or pancreatic duct
5. Sphincterotomy
6. Endoscopic intervention:
   a. Stent placement
   b. Balloon or basket extraction of biliary stones
   c. Laser lithotripsy

The AGA standards for office-based GI endoscopy were written in response to market changes in physician reimbursements for many endoscopic procedures that will continue to drive their performance into unregulated office-based setting. On the basis of the desire to maximize patient safety, the following list of procedures and conditions was compiled to limit situations in which patients would be put at risk (see Box 13.7).

Box 13.7 • Procedures Not To Be Undertaken in the Office Setting

1. Stent placement ERCP
2. Endoscopic sphincterotomy
3. Endoscopic ultrasound with pseudocyst drainage
4. Removal of suspected foreign body
5. Endoscopic management of gastroesophageal reflux disease
6. Therapeutic hemostatic control of acute bleeding
7. Procedures deemed emergent
8. Procedures carrying a considerable risk of bleeding or major complications

---

COMPLICATIONS

Bleeding, perforation of hollow structures, infection, and problems related to conscious sedation are complications that can be seen. Complications during GI endoscopy result mostly from interventional procedures. Hemorrhage following polypectomy is frequently seen and is managed endoscopically, but may require surgical intervention. Perforation during colonoscopy can lead to a distended abdomen with venous compromise and hemodynamic responses due to decreased preload. Variceal bleeding can lead to significant blood loss, which may lead to circulatory compromise and death.

This emphasizes the need for health care personnel skilled in airway management and emergency resuscitative techniques to be present or immediately available should any problem arise.

REFERENCES

1. Seeff LC, Richards TB, Shapiro JA, et al. How many endoscopies are performed for colorectal cancer screening? Results from CDC's survey of endoscopic capacity. *Gastroenterology*. 2004;127:1670–1677.
2. Faigel DO, Baron TH, Goldstein JL, et al. Guidelines for the use of deep sedation and anesthesia for GI endoscopy. *Gastrointest Endosc*. 2002;56:613–617.
3. American Society for Gastrointestinal Endoscopy. Training guideline for use of propofol in gastrointestinal endoscopy. *Gastrointest Endosc*. 2004; 60:167–172.
4. Waring JP, Baron TH, Hirota WK, et al. Guidelines for conscious sedation and monitoring during gastrointestinal endoscopy. *Gastrointest Endosc*. 2003;58:317–322.
5. Benjamin SB. Complications of conscious sedation. *Gastrointest Endosc Clin N Am*. 1996;6:277–286.
6. Freeman ML. Sedation and monitoring for gastrointestinal endoscopy. *Gastrointest Endosc Clin N Am*. 1994;4:475–499.
7. Quine MA, Bell GD, McCloy RF, et al. Prospective audit of upper gastrointestinal endoscopy in two regions of England: Safety, staffing, and sedation methods. *Gut*. 1995;36:462–467.
8. Arrowsmith JB, Gerstman BB, Fleischer DE, et al. Results from the American Society for Gastrointestinal Endoscopy/U.S. Food and Drug Administration collaborative study on complication rates and drug use during gastrointestinal endoscopy. *Gastrointest Endosc*. 1991;37:421–427.

9. Heuss LT, Schnieper P, Drewe J, et al. Safety of propofol for conscious sedation during endoscopic procedures in high-risk patients-a prospective, controlled study. *Am J Gastroenterol.* 2003;98:1751–1757.

10. Heuss LT, Schnieper P, Drewe J, et al. Conscious sedation with propofol in elderly patients: A prospective evaluation. *Aliment Pharmacol Ther.* 2003;17: 1493–1501.

11. Goff JS. Effect of propofol on human sphincter of Oddi. *Dig Dis Sci.* 1995;40:2364–2367.

12. Walker JA, McIntyre RD, Schleinitz PF, et al. Nurse-administered propofol sedation without anesthesia specialists in 9152 endoscopic cases in an ambulatory surgery center. *Am J Gastroenterol.* 2003;98:1744–1750.

13. Koshy G, Nair S, Norkus EP, et al. Propofol versus midazolam and meperidine for conscious sedation in GI endoscopy. *Am J Gastroenterol.* 2000;95: 1476–1479.

14. Jung M, Hofmann C, Kiesslich R, et al. Improved sedation in diagnostic and therapeutic ERCP: Propofol is an alternative to midazolam. *Endoscopy.* 2000;32:233–238.

15. Rex DK, Overley C, Kinser K, et al. Safety of propofol administered by registered nurses with gastroenterologist supervision in 2000 endoscopic cases. *Am J Gastroenterol.* 2002;97:1159–1163.

16. Seifert H, Schmitt TH, Gultekin T, et al. Sedation with propofol plus midazolam versus propofol alone for interventional endoscopic procedures: A prospective, randomized study. *Aliment Pharmacol Ther.* 2000;14:1207–1214.

17. Sipe BW, Rex DK, Latinovich D, et al. Propofol versus midazolam/meperidine for outpatient colonoscopy: Administration by nurses supervised by endoscopists. *Gastrointest Endosc.* 2002;55:815–825.

18. Vargo JJ, Zuccaro G Jr, Dumot JA, et al. Gastroenterologist-administered propofol for therapeutic upper endoscopy with graphic assessment of respiratory activity: A case series. *Gastrointest Endosc.* 2000;52:250–255.

19. Vargo JJ, Zuccaro G Jr, Dumot JA, et al. Gastroenterologist-administered propofol versus meperidine and midazolam for advanced upper endoscopy: A prospective, randomized trial. *Gastroenterology.* 2002;123:8–16.

20. Wehrmann T, Kokabpick S, Lembcke B, et al. Efficacy and safety of intravenous propofol sedation during routine ERCP: A prospective, controlled study. *Gastrointest Endosc.* 1999;49:677–683.

21. Crantock L, Cowen AE, Ward M, et al. Supplemental low flow oxygen prevents hypoxia during endoscopic cholangiopancreatography. *Gastrointest Endosc.* 1992;38:418–420.

22. Reshef R, Shiller M, Kinberg R, et al. A prospective study evaluating the usefulness of continuous supplemental oxygen in various endoscopic procedures. *Isr J Med Sci.* 1996;32:736–740.

23. Nelson DB, Freeman ML, Silvis SE, et al. A randomized, controlled trial of transcutaneous carbon dioxide monitoring during ERCP. *Gastrointest Endosc.* 2000;51:288–295.

24. Fu ES, Downs JB, Schweiger JW, et al. Supplemental oxygen impairs detection of hypoventilation by pulse oximetry. *Chest.* 2004;126:1552–1558.

25. Soto RG, Fu ES, Vila H Jr, et al. Capnography accurately detects apnea during monitored anesthesia care. *Anesth Analg.* 2004;99:379–382.

26. Vargo JJ, Zuccaro G Jr, Dumot JA, et al. Automated graphic assessment of respiratory activity is superior to pulse oximetry and visual assessment for the detection of early respiratory depression during therapeutic upper endoscopy. *Gastrointest Endosc.* 2002;55:826–831.

27. Bower AL, Ripepi A, Dilger J, et al. Bispectral index monitoring of sedation during endoscopy. *Gastrointest Endosc.* 2000;52:192–196.

28. Lazzaroni M, Bianchi Porro G. Preparation, premedication, and surveillance. *Endoscopy*. 2005;37:101–109.

29. Chernik DA, Gillings D, Laine H, et al. Validity and reliability of the observer's assessment of alertness/sedation scale: Study with intravenous midazolam. *J Clin Psychopharmacol*. 1990;10:244–251.

30. The American Gastroenterological Association. The American Gastroenterological Association standards for office-based gastrointestinal endoscopy services. *Gastroenterology*. 2001;121(2):440–443.

Post-Bariatric Surgery: A New Body Contour

Stephanie A. Caterson, Karinne Jervis, and
Richard D. Urman

Obesity is an increasingly important health care epidemic in the United States affecting approximately 23% of the adult population who have a body mass index (BMI) >30. Five percent of Americans are estimated to be morbidly obese (BMI ≥ 40). General morbidity and mortality are increased in obese patients and life expectancy may be reduced by as much as 20 years. Obesity has many associated comorbidities, many of which are reversed with weight loss (see Box 14.1).

Box 14.1

Comorbidities Associated with Obesity
- Hypertension
- Coronary artery disease
- Cardiomyopathy
- Pulmonary hypertension
- Cholecystitis/cholelithiasis
- Reflux esophagitis
- Obstructive sleep apnea
- Diabetes mellitus, type 2
- High cholesterol
- Depression
- Anovulation
- Intertrigo
- Venous varicosities
- Chronic back, neck, knee, and foot pain
- Increased operative risk

Weight loss techniques vary from straightforward diet and exercise to more invasive surgical interventions. Bariatric surgery is reserved for patients who have failed to lose weight through conventional means. Multiple bariatric surgical procedures have been developed including laparoscopic gastric banding and gastric bypass. Advances in surgical techniques, along with a rising public interest, have resulted in an approximately 600% increase in gastric bypass surgeries between 1998 and 2002. A gastric bypass effectively reduces the capacity of the stomach, resulting in an earlier sensation of satiety. The large extent of weight loss is secondary to a reduction in food intake with typical results averaging 69% to 82% of excess weight lost over 12 to 54 months.

Regardless of the weight reduction method, massive weight loss (MWL) results in major changes for the patient that are both physiologic and aesthetic. These patients have been shown to have a reduction in their presurgical comorbidities as well as an increase in self-esteem, body image, and eating behaviors. Unfortunately there are some side effects from both the gastric surgery and the MWL (see Table 14.1). Many obese patients lose skin elasticity due to the persistent stretching of the skin as their body

Table 14.1. Massive weight loss advantages and disadvantages

Advantages	Disadvantages
Decrease in medical comorbidities	Excess loose/folding skin
Increased self esteem/body image	Nutritional deficits
Improved eating habits	Anemia
	Potential surgical complications

surface area increases. After MWL, the skin is often incapable of retraction and there are resultant areas of redundant skin. Personal hygiene and skin infection—related issues, along with desire for improved body contour, often result in a plastic surgical consultation. Many body contour procedures are offered by plastic surgeons, most of which can be done in an appropriate office setting. Plastic surgeons aim for multiple goals with body contour surgery, listed in Box 14.2. Because of the poor quality and large quantity of redundant tissue, the goals of surgery often cannot be achieved with liposuction alone, and usually require direct excision of tissue.

Box 14.2

Goals of Body Contouring Surgery
- Removal of excess/redundant skin and fat
- Anatomic repositioning of gravitationally affected parts
- Re-establishing normal body forms and curves

In 2006, the American Society of Plastic Surgeons (ASPS) reported more than 68,000 body contour cases performed on MWL patients during the previous year. There was a 22% increase in body contouring cases when compared with 2004. This number is targeted to increase dramatically as gastric bypass surgery becomes more readily available. Of all cosmetic procedures performed by plastic surgeons, 62% are office based and 17% occur in a freestanding ambulatory surgical facility. The remaining 21% are performed in a hospital. Offering cosmetic procedures in the office can dramatically decrease the cost associated with the procedure for the patient, but it must be performed safely with appropriate anesthetic intervention.

Several issues must be considered before an MWL patient is brought to surgery (see Box 14.3). First, careful attention is made to the patient's nutritional status. Many gastric bypass patients have B_{12} deficiency, anemia, hypocalcemia, and other deficiencies. Second, surgeons require a 6- to 12-month stable weight after MWL has occurred to allow for reduction in obesity-related comorbidities. Finally, most patients are interested in addressing several areas of the body to complete their contour procedures. Because of the length and complexity of the operations, the anesthesiologist and the plastic surgeon need to work closely to decide how much surgery to pursue in a single stage. Increased operative time will subject the patient to additional hypothermia, blood loss, fluid shifts, and risk of blood clots. Often, a complete body contouring process is divided into several operations for the sake of safety (see Figure 14.1). Careful preoperative assessment of the airway is especially important in MWL patients, some of which may have a history of severe sleep apnea or gastric reflux.

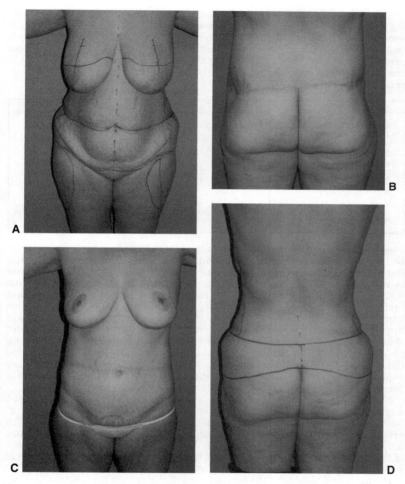

Figure 14.1.   A and B represent an image of a patient about to undergo several operations for body contouring. C and D represent the outcome.

Box 14.3

Safety Considerations of the Preoperative Massive Weight Loss Patient
- Nutritional status
- Stable weight pattern
- Status of comorbidities
- Multiple body parts to be addressed—consider staging procedures
- Airway assessment

As previously mentioned, multiple surgical options exist for body contouring (see Box 14.4). These procedures are not trivial and usually require a general anesthetic and a significant recovery period. Cautious patient positioning in the operating room is essential. Often the patient is moved from prone to supine (or vice versa) during the procedure. Judicious protection of the airway must be maintained as well as prudent pressure relief of bony prominences.

Box 14.4

Common Body Contouring Procedures
- Abdominoplasty
- Lower body lift
- Mastopexy/augmentation
- Upper body lift
- Brachioplasty
- Thigh lift
- Face/neck lift

Abdominoplasty is the most commonly performed body contouring surgery. During this procedure the lower abdominal skin and fat are removed, leaving the umbilicus attached as a stalk. The rectus muscles are plicated if there is a diastasis, and the upper abdominal skin is pulled down. The resultant scars go from hip to hip along the inguinal and suprapubic regions and around the umbilicus. Abdominoplasty may be combined successfully with suction-assisted lipoplasty if obstinate collections of fat remain. A lower body lift, also known as a *belt lipectomy*, involves similar wedge resections of skin and fat of the lower back/upper buttock area in conjunction with the abdominoplasty. The resultant scar continues around the back just above the superior buttocks. This procedure requires the patient to be turned from supine to prone while under anesthesia, often more than once. This careful positioning significantly increases operative time.

Mastopexy, or breast lift, can be performed with or without implant augmentation. Here, the nipple/areolar complex is lifted to a more youthful position, and excess breast skin is removed. Resultant scars are around the areola, and may continue vertically to the inframammary fold (IMF) and horizontally along the IMF. An upper body lift addresses the skin and fat of the upper back and thorax. Similar to the lower body lift, excess tissue is removed and a curvilinear scar remains across the back.

During a brachioplasty, the excess tissue of the upper arm is removed in an elliptical manner, with ensuing scars that run parallel to the extremity on the medial upper arm from axilla to elbow. A thigh lift can be performed through an elliptical incision that parallels the inguinal crease inferiorly. Sometimes a vertical component is required that leaves a resultant scar along the medial thigh. It can be challenging for the anesthesiologist to provide peripheral intravenous access if brachioplasty is combined with a thigh lift. One can move the line access during the case to avoid the surgical fields, or consider alternative access routes such as the external jugular vein or central venous access.

Finally, MWL patients can also develop excess sagging of the face and neck skin that can be managed with traditional face and neck lift approaches. Usual scars run from the temporal hair bearing area, in front of and behind the ear, and onto the posterior scalp. Also, a submental incision is often made to attend to the excess neck skin.

In reality, no two patients are exactly the same, and this is particularly true of the body contouring population following bariatric surgery and subsequent weight loss. Usually a combination of several of the procedures listed in the preceding text can be performed during a single sitting. Exactly how much surgery can be performed is not clearly defined in the literature. Guidelines for utilizing multiple experienced surgical teams and limiting operative times to approximately 5 to 6 hours have been suggested.

The MWL patient group in particular is subject to a laundry list of potential complications (see Box 14.5). Because of the massive skin exposure required in the operating room, hypothermia is very common. Blood loss can be masked due to large skin flap elevation and multiple positional shifts during the case. Attention should be given to maintaining normothermia and replacing blood products as needed. Aggressive prophylaxis to prevent blood clots is imperative. Although opinions vary on exact protocols, individual institutions should develop guidelines for MWL body contour patients that are agreeable to the plastic surgeon and the anesthesiologist. Because of the large skin flaps that are raised during the operation, postoperative hematoma and seroma are all too common. Surgical drains are used in almost every case. Also, the MWL patient is prone to wound healing complications, infections, and unfavorable scarring. The causes of these are multifactorial, and can be optimized by careful preoperative assessment of the specific issues associated with MWL patients (Box 14.3).

Box 14.5

Complications Encountered in the Massive Weight Loss Patient
- Intraoperative hypothermia
- Intraoperative blood loss
- Fluid shifts
- deep vein thrombosis (DVT)/pulmonary embolism(PE)
- Hematoma
- Seroma
- Unfavorable scarring
- Wound healing problems
- Infections

Complications arising from surgeries performed in an office setting led to a moratorium on procedures in Florida, requiring general anesthetic and heavy sedation in 2002. The 90- day moratorium placed on office-based practices was due to an increased risk of mortality from 1 in 47,215 (with liposuction alone) to 1 in 3,281 (with a combined liposuction and abdominoplasty). In the MWL patient, the anesthesiologist must be cognizant of the patient's comorbidity, multiple procedures, length of surgery, and *use of tumescent fluids for liposuction. The patient may experience massive fluid shifts dependant on total volume of wetting solution used to infiltrate the subcutaneous tissue (50%–70% of infiltrated volume is presumed to be intravascular), total amount of lipoaspirate (fluid plus fat removed), and the total amount of local anesthetic concentrations*. In 2004 the ASPS committee on patient safety announced a practice advisory on liposuction that recommended limiting the amount of lidocaine in the tumescent solution to 35 mg per kg and removing no more than 5,000 mL of lipoaspirate. This is usually not a concern in the MWL patient, as liposuction plays a limited role due to poor skin elasticity.

Postoperatively, the anesthesiologist must be aware of potential cardiac and pulmonary complications related to the primary surgical procedure, local anesthetic concentrations, fluid shifts, temperature regulation, anesthetic agents, narcotics, and pain. In some institutions, the plastic surgeons can utilize a "pain pump" for postoperative pain management consisting of a sustained low volume release of local anesthetic through a catheter placed in the subcutaneous position.

SUGGESTED READINGS

Iverson RE, Lynch DJ. The ASPS Committee on Patient Safety. Practice advisory on liposuction. *Plast Reconstr Surg*. 2004;113(5): 1478–1490.

Safety considerations and avoiding complications in the massive weight loss patient. Body contouring after massive weight loss. *Plast Reconstr Surg*. 2006;117(1 suppl): 74S–81S.

Smoot TM, Xu P, Hilsenrath P, et al. Gastric bypass surgery in the United States, 1998–2002. *Am J Public Health*. 2006;96: 1187–1189.

Pain

Cristin A. McMurray

Pain is a complex process influenced by physiologic and psychologic factors. It is estimated that in 2005, approximately 80% of all surgeries were performed on an outpatient basis. Surveys indicate that 80% of patients experience moderate to severe pain postoperatively (1). This is an astounding number considering the advancements in technology regarding drug delivery systems and the improved number and type of medications for pain relief that are available.

WHY DO WE CARE ABOUT PAIN?

In addition to the basic humanitarian desire to alleviate pain in patients, there are actually a number of important consequences to postoperative pain in the ambulatory setting (see Box 15.1). The experience of pain has numerous effects on various organ systems throughout the body that can develop into problematic sequellae for patients. Most notably in the postoperative setting, pain may lead *to splinting and reduced cough*. These conditions, in turn, lead to *atelectasis and hypoxemia*. Pain also *increases myocardial oxygen demand*, which, in combination with the aforementioned hypoxemia, could expose the heart to ischemia. Pain affects the gastrointestinal (GI) system by *reducing motility and gastric emptying*, which can *increase nausea and vomiting*. Additionally, pain can cause *urinary retention, hyperglycemia, and anxiety*. The reduced mobility from pain may expose the patient to the risk of pressure sores and possible *deep vein thrombosis or pulmonary embolism* (2). All of these problems may lead to longer postanesthesia care unit (PACU) stays and possible unanticipated hospital admissions; it makes medical as well as financial sense to optimize pain control in the outpatient setting. Recent Joint Commission on Accreditation of Healthcare Organizations (JCAHO) guidelines stress the importance of pain assessment (also known as the *fifth* vital sign), good multidisciplinary pain management, patient education, and monitoring the performance of the health care team in carrying out these guidelines.

Box 15.1

Physiologic Effect of Pain
Splinting and reduced cough
Atelectasis and hypoxemia
Increase in myocardial oxygen demand
Reduced gastric motility and emptying
Increased nausea and vomiting
Urinary retention
Hyperglycemia
Anxiety

Historically, physicians are noted to have undertreated pain; fear of causing respiratory depression leads many clinicians to undertreat pain. The goal should be a balance, or perhaps a better understanding of the way that pain affects patients and ways that patients affect their own pain perceptions. With the array of drugs in the therapeutic arsenal, a little empathy and openness to some "alternative" modalities of pain modulation, anesthesiologists can make a difference to patients and the impact pain has in the postoperative period.

A BIOPSYCHOSOCIAL MODEL OF PAIN

Understanding the ways in which pain affects patients is extremely important, even for what are considered, "minor" surgeries in an office setting. As clinicians have less time to spend with these patients than in a hospital setting, it is crucial to be able to anticipate patients' responses to pain they may undergo. The biopsychosocial model of pain serves to elucidate some of the factors that may not come immediately to mind if one regards pain as a purely physical state. This *sensory component* is certainly important, but there are other aspects to consider (see Box 15.2). There are *emotional, cognitive, behavioral, environmental, and social factors* involved with an individual's response to pain. In the acute setting, the psychosocial components are probably more relevant, but many patients coming for surgery may have issues with chronic pain (see Box 15.3).

Box 15.2 • The Biopsychosocial Model of Pain

Sensory component
Emotional component
Cognitive aspects
Behavioral factors
Environmental and social factors

Box 15.3 • Patient Issues Affecting Anesthesia

Loss of control
Feelings of helplessness
May exacerbate pain

Another issue for many patients undergoing anesthesia for surgery is a *loss of control*; *feelings of helplessness* may also accompany their postoperative pain experience and *exacerbate their pain*. Physicians should try to remain aware of patients' individual experiences and try to tailor their interpersonal and medical treatment accordingly (3).

PHARMACOLOGIC TREATMENT OF PAIN

There are various models illustrating basic principles in treating acute pain. The World Health Organization (WHO) and World Federation of Societies of Anesthesiologists (WFSA) have both created "Analgesic Ladders" to help providers think about how to approach pain.

The WHO Analgesic Ladder (see Figure 15.1) was introduced to improve pain control in patients with cancer pain. It also educates the practitioner regarding the management of acute pain as it employs a logical strategy to pain management. As originally described, the ladder has three rungs.

The WFSA Analgesic Ladder (see Figure 15.2) has been developed to treat acute pain. Initially, the pain can be expected to be severe and may need controlling with strong analgesics in combination with local anesthetic blocks and peripherally acting drugs (4).

LOCAL ANESTHETICS

A small amount of local anesthesia can go a long way in preventing severe postoperative pain. It can be administered for the actual surgery itself, and, if properly maintained in the postoperative period, may serve as the major component of pain management for a patient. This may be extremely beneficial in patients whose respiratory and cardiac status may not be ideal.

Local anesthetics work to prevent depolarization in nerve cell membranes by inhibiting sodium channels. There are a number of local anesthetic drugs

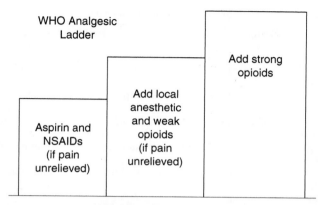

Figure 15.1. The World Health Organization (WHO) Analgesic Ladder. NSAIDs, nonsteroidal anti-inflammatory drugs.

available which differ in their duration of action and toxicity profiles (see Table 15.1).

In the ambulatory setting, local can be used in a variety of ways by both surgeons and anesthesiologists.

The most basic use for local is infiltration of the wound, usually done by surgeons, either before, during, or after the surgery. Sometimes this might be all that the patient requires. In other instances, the addition of intravenous (IV) sedation may serve to help the patient tolerate the local infiltration and the procedure itself. Other times, the surgeons may inject local anesthetic at the end of a general anesthetic to help with postoperative pain. Ideally the local anesthetic would serve to maintain the patient during the immediate postoperative course until other pain control methods could begin to work. Interestingly, there are current studies on continuous wound infusion pumps that administer local anesthetics; results have been mixed, but there is

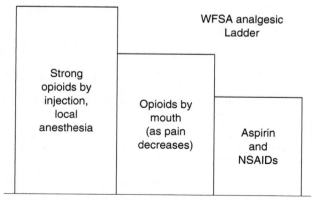

Figure 15.2. The World Federation of Societies of Anesthesiologists (WFSA) Analgesic Ladder. NSAIDs, nonsteroidal anti-inflammatory drugs.

Table 15.1.   Local anesthetic doses and properties

Medication	Maximum dose (with epi)	Onset	Duration (with epi)
Bupivacaine (Marcaine)	2.5 mg/kg (3 mg/kg)	Slow	4 h (8 h)
Etidocaine (Duranest)	2.5 mg/kg (4 mg/kg)	Rapid	4 h (8 h)
Lidocaine (Xylocaine)	4.5 mg/kg (7 mg/kg)	Rapid	120 min (240 min)
Mepivacaine (Carbocaine)	4.5 mg/kg (7 mg/kg)	Rapid	180 min (360 min)
Prilocaine (Citanest)	5 mg/kg (7.5 mg/kg)	Medium	90 min (360 min)
Ropivacaine	3 mg/kg	Rapid–Medium	2–6 h
Chloroprocaine (Nesacaine)	10 mg/kg (15 mg/kg)	Rapid	30 min (90 min)
Procaine	8 mg/kg (10 mg/kg)	Slow	45 min (90 min)
Tetracaine (Pontocaine)	1.5 mg/kg (2.5 mg/kg)	Slow	3 h (10 h)

evidence that they may be as effective as patient-controlled anesthesia (PCA) for some types of postoperative pain (1).

REGIONAL ANESTHETICS

Regional anesthesia is the fairly self-explanatory name for anesthetizing areas of the body, allowing surgery to be performed without the use of general anesthesia (GA). Alternately, a regional block may be employed in conjunction with GA either to reduce the need for narcotics or to help with postoperative pain. Local anesthetic, with or without adjuvant medications (e.g., opioids, epinephrine, bicarbonate, clonidine) is injected close to the nerves innervating the surgical field. Many times a nerve stimulator is useful to help localize the correct nerve. Sensory nerves (with their smaller size and more peripheral location in the neural bundle), are anesthetized first, followed by the motor nerves. It is fortunate in terms of PACU time-to-discharge that motor nerves are the first to return; patients are able to ambulate and can be discharged home with good sensory analgesia that remains postoperatively (see Table 15.2).

Regional blocks may be administered as single-shot injections either alone or in conjunction with other single injections to anesthetize a larger area or extremity. *Paravertebral blocks* have regained interest for their use in *breast surgery*, and the combination of *lumbar plexus, femoral, and sciatic blocks for total knee replacements* seems to be vying in popularity with neuraxial blockade for these surgeries (1). Continuous regional catheters may also be inserted into larger nerve sheaths to provide infusions of local. In the ambulatory setting, this could be best served in the upper extremities. Patient-controlled regional anesthetic pumps that the patients are sent home with might be an innovative way to control postoperative pain for ambulatory patients (5). There has been exciting work done with wounded soldiers whose combat-related pain has been managed with such pumps for their transit back to hospitals (6) (see Table 15.3 and Box 15.4).

Table 15.2. Appropriate nerve block technique selection

Nerve Block	Type of Surgery
Interscalene block	Shoulder, arm, and elbow surgery
Infraclavicular block	Elbow, forearm, and hand surgery
Axillary block	Forearm and hand surgery, if surgery does not require prolonged tourniquet time
Wrist/digital blocks	Surgery of hand and fingers if no tourniquet required for surgery
Intravenous regional block (Bier's block)	Surgery of wrist, hand, or fingers
Femoral nerve block	Surgery of anterior thigh and knee (if combined with genitofemoral block can be used for saphenous vein stripping)
Sciatic nerve block	Surgery of knee, tibia, ankle, or foot
Popliteal block	Surgery of ankle, foot, short saphenous vein stripping

Box 15.4

Basic Supplies for Nerve Blocks
Monitoring equipment such as automated blood pressure, pulse oximetry, and electrocardiograph
Emergency airway equipment
(Oxygen supply, Ambu-bag, suction, laryngoscopy handles/blades, styletted endotracheal tubes)
Emergency drugs
(ephedrine, atropine, phenylephrine, epinephrine, midazolam, propofol, succinylcholine, intralipid)
Insulated needles in several sizes (50 mm, 100 mm)—experts recommend short bevel, blunt needles
Nerve stimulator
Ancillary supplies such as syringes, needles, stopcocks, alcohol swabs, gauze, skin marking pens

Neuraxial anesthesia is another important use of local anesthetic, again, with or without adjuncts such as epinephrine or opioids. Spinal, epidural, and caudal blocks can all be used for anesthesia for surgery and for postoperative pain. In the office or ambulatory setting, intrathecal blockade is more frequently utilized than other neuraxial methods due to its reliability and quick onset of action. Single-shot epidural techniques and caudal techniques are not often performed in adults due to their unpredictable nature and the delayed time until the block sets up. Continuous epidural catheters are not often used for outpatients unless there is a compelling reason not to use a spinal, and obviously the catheter must be removed before the patient is discharged (1).

SYSTEMIC DRUGS AND THEIR DELIVERY
Anesthesiologists use various methods and routes of administration for delivery of medications to treat pain. The IV route is used perioperatively and in the PACU; upon discharge patients must be transitioned to oral medications. In most ambulatory patients, IV and PO medications are the norm,

Table 15.3. Nerve blocks at a glance

Nerve Block	Nerve Stimulator Current	Desired Response	Local Anesthetic (example common drug)
Interscalene (brachial plexus block)	0.2–0.4 mA	Twitch of pectoralis, deltoid, arm, forearm, or hand muscles	35–40 mL (bupivacaine 0.5% + epi)
Infraclavicular (brachial plexus block)	0.2–0.3 mA	Hand twitch (preferably median nerve)	30–45 mL (mepivacaine 1.5% + HCO$_3$ + epi)
Axillary (brachial plexus block)	0.2–0.4 mA	Hand twitch (if aspirate blood, acceptable to use axillary artery as landmark)	35–40 mL (mepivacaine 1.5% + HCO$_3$ + epi)
Sciatic (sciatic nerve block)	0.2–0.5 mA	Twitch of hamstring, calf, foot, or toes	20 mL (mepivacaine 1.5% + HCO$_3$)
Femoral (femoral nerve block)	0.2–0.5 mA	Patellar twitch (quadriceps)	20 mL (Mepivacaine 1.5% + HCO$_3$ + epi)
Popliteal (sciatic nerve block at popliteal fossa)	0.2–0.5 mA	Twitch of foot or toes	35–45 mL (Mepivacaine 1.5% + HCO$_3$ + epi)

(Adapted from Hadzic A, Vloka J. *Peripheral nerve blocks: Principles and practice.* New York: McGraw-Hill; 2004.)

but remember that there are also alternate routes, such as intramuscular (IM), nasal, rectal, sublingual, and transdermal, that may be beneficial in selected individuals.

CLASSES OF ANALGESIC DRUGS

Broadly speaking, pain medications can be divided into opioids and nonopioids. Opioid use tends to be effective in the perioperative setting, but studies (and the WHO step-ladder approach) have shown that combinations of medicines are more effective than single medications alone (1).

ACETAMINOPHEN

Tylenol has analgesic and antipyretic effects, without anti-inflammatory effects. Acetaminophen can be given orally or rectally. It is often already combined with opioids (e.g., oxycodone and hydrocodone) for prescription and administration, but it can also be useful on its own. Metabolism is through the liver, and the maximum daily dose is 4 g. Normally the cytochrome P-450 pathway only converts a small percentage of acetaminophen to a toxic metabolite. The consumption of alcohol, however, induces greater expression of the cytochrome P-450 pathway and may lead to increased levels of this toxic metabolite (N-acetyl-p-benzoquinone imine) in the body. It may be wise to reduce maximum doses of acetaminophen to 2 g per day for those patients with a history of significant alcohol consumption or patients with liver problems (4).

NONSTEROIDAL ANTI-INFLAMMATORY DRUGS

Nonsteroidal anti-inflammatory drugs (NSAIDs) can be extremely useful for postoperative pain (see Box 15.5 and Table 15.4). Their anti-inflammatory and analgesic effects help with tissue swelling and pain. They work by inhibiting cyclo-oxygenase (COX) enzymes, which, in turn, inhibits the production of prostaglandins, prostacyclins, and thromboxane (see Box 15.6). Prostaglandins PGE2 and PGI2 are normally increased during inflammation and sensitize the pain-transmitting C fibers to the pain neurotransmitters.

> **Box 15.5**
>
> There are several different kinds of NSAIDs available over the counter such as aspirin, ibuprofen, and naproxen. There are also other oral NSAIDs that are available by prescription. The only parenteral NSAID currently available is ketorolac. There are also topical and suppository formulations for some NSAIDs, which may be useful in select patients. All NSAIDs operate by the same mechanism; however, an individual's response to each may vary. NSAIDs seem to work particularly well for pain emerging from skin, buccal mucosa, joint surfaces, and bone (4). In the office-based setting, NSAIDs may most commonly be used in a similar sequence as other medications, transitioning from IV to PO administration. Owing to the potential side effects, caution should be exercised in patients with known GI, renal, or hematologic disorders.

> **Box 15.6 • Possible Effects of COX-1 Inhibition**
>
> - Increased risk of GI bleeding
> - Decreased renal plasma flow and decreased GFR
> - Disturbances in platelet aggregation

Side effects such as platelet dysfunction may lead to increased postoperative bleeding. Patients should be cautioned about the potential gastric side

Table 15.4. Typical nonopioid analgesics and doses

Medication	Dose	Onset of Action	Duration of Action
Aspirin	500—1,000 mg PO q 4—6 h	30–60 min	4 h
Acetaminophen	500—1,000 mg PO q 4–6 h (max 4 gm/24 h)	30 min	4 h
Ibuprofen	400–800 PO q 4—8 h	30 min	4–6 h
Naproxen sodium	Naproxen sodium 275—550 mg PO q 8–12 h	1–2 h	8–12 h
Ketorolac	IV/IM: 15–30 mg q 6 h PO: 10 mg q 4–6 h	IV/IM: 10–60 min PO: 30–60 min	4–6 h (recommend use only for 5 d)

effects of oral NSAIDs, especially in conjunction with heavy alcohol use. Both alcohol and NSAID use place patients at higher risk for upper GI bleeding; this risk is magnified if patients consume both. Remember that NSAIDs inhibit COX-1, which decreases mucus and bicarbonate, lowers mucosal blood flow, and inhibits epithelial proliferation; this effect, along with additional effects on platelet aggregation, can lead to bleeding in the GI tract. Also, remember that ketorolac and other NSAIDs may be problematic in patients with renal dysfunction; COX-1 is responsible for producing vasodilating prostaglandins to maintain renal plasma flow and glomerular filtration rate (GFR). In the presence of NSAIDs this mechanism fails and may expose the already compromised kidney to more damage. Although NSAIDs are excellent medication for the treatment of acute postoperative pain, their use must be carefully considered in all cases; any concerns should be discussed with the surgeon in advance.

OPIOIDS

Opioids are an anesthesiologist's mainstay treatment for pain. Opioids bind to receptors in the central nervous system (CNS), as well as receptors in the somatic and sympathetic peripheral nerves. Activation of the μ, δ and κ receptors causes a decrease of signal transmission from the primary peripheral afferent neurons to the CNS. Individual drugs differ in their affinity for the various subtypes of receptors, which account for their differences in efficacy and side effects. The main side effects are respiratory depression, nausea, and vomiting. Currently there are oral, IV, IM, sublingual, transdermal, and rectal formulations available (see Table 15.5). As with most other drugs in the perioperative period, it is most practical to begin with the IV route and transition the patient to the oral route after surgery for home use (1).

In the office-based setting, with patients who will be discharged home shortly after their surgeries, it is prudent to use short-acting IV narcotics such as fentanyl, alfentanil, sufentanil, or remifentanil. Morphine, hydromorphone (Dilaudid), and meperidine (Demerol) have longer half-lives (ranging from 2–4 hours) and their side effects may be longer than predicted. This can cause an increase in PACU time and can increase the patient's chances for an unanticipated hospital admission. Although these drugs can certainly be

Table 15.5. Typical opioid analgesics and doses

Medication	Dose	Onset of Action	Duration of Action
Acetaminophen 325 mg/codeine 300 mg (Tylenol No. 3)	1–2 tablets PO q 4–6 h	30–45 min	4–6 h
Fentanyl	0.5–1.5 μg/kg IV (usually 50–100 μg)	1–3 min	30–60 min
Hydrocodone 5 mg/ acetaminophen 500 mg (Vicodin)	1–2 tablets PO q 4–6 h (5–10 mg hydrocodone)	10–30 min	4–6 h
Hydromorphone (Dilaudid)	IV: 0.2—1 mg q 3 h	IV: 4–6 min	IV: 2—3 h
	IM: 1–2 mg q 4–6 h	IM: 10–15 min	IM: 4–5 h
	PO: 2 mg q 3–6 h	PO: 30 min	PO: 4 h
Morphine (immediate release)	IV/SC: 1–10 mg q 2–4 h	IV: 4-–6 min	4–5 h for all routes
	IM: 5–20 mg q 4 h	IM: 10–30 min	
	PO: 10–30 mg q 4 h	PO: 30–60 min	
Morphine (sustained release)	10–30 mg PO q 8–12 h	30–60 min	3–8 h
Meperidine (Demerol) Not recommended except for treatment of rigors	25–50 mg IV for rigors	1 min	24 h
Oxycodone (immediate release)	5–15 mg PO q 4–6 h	—	3–4 h
Oxycodone (sustained release)	10 mg PO q 12 h	30—60 min	12 h
Oxycodone 5 mg/ acetaminophen 325 mg (Percocet)	1–2 tablets PO q 4–6 h	10–30 min	3–6 h
Propoxyphene 65 mg/ acetaminophen 650 mg (Darvocet)	1 tablet PO q 4–6 h	15–60 min	4–6 h
Methadone (Dolophine)	IV/SC: 2.5–10 mg	PO: 30–60 min	4–6 h
	PO: 5–20 mg q 6–8 h		

used for ambulatory patients, their use should be well planned with the added recovery time considered.

Initially in the PACU, IV medication can be utilized; usually the transition to oral medications should be relatively quick. Once the patient is able to tolerate PO, the oral route will be longer acting. If they exhibit any side effects such as nausea, vomiting, or respiratory depression, they should be assessed before discharge. One drawback to oral medication at this point is that absorption may be delayed secondary to postoperative delays in gastric emptying, as well as postoperative nausea and vomiting (PONV).

For minor pain, codeine, with or without acetaminophen, can be useful for patients. The most commonly prescribed postoperative pain medications are hydrocodone and oxycodone in combination with acetaminophen. These are often well tolerated; however, patients may require concurrent antiemetics. Meperidine and propoxyphene (alone or with acetaminophen) are also possible choices for postoperative pain. A simple rule of thumb: *It is helpful to ask patients what medicines they have used in the past that have been successful in treating pain and if they have had particular failure with certain drugs.*

CONCLUSIONS

Postoperative pain is important to recognize and treat, especially in ambulatory patients who will be monitored for a short time in the PACU and discharged home within a few hours. Narcotic-sparing techniques utilizing local anesthetics can assist patients in reducing pain. When used in combination, the dose of each can be decreased, thereby decreasing their potential side effects. Combinations of opioids and NSAIDs, when indicated, can often work better than opioids alone. Regardless of the setting, the best treatment for postoperative pain is to have a well thought-out plan in advance, tailored to individual patient needs.

If the optimal goal of the office-based setting is to provide a safe and pleasant experience, anesthesiologists need to recognize the importance of providing patients with both physical and emotional comfort; "TLC" (a little tender loving care) can be equally as important as administering medications. Evidence to support this concept was shown in Henry Beecher's classic article about the significance of the "placebo effect.". In his early study, he documented how both physiologic and psychological changes could be seen in patients, solely due to a placebo (7).

The informed public is seeking alternative and nonpharmacologic means to help with pain and anxiety; these techniques will be discussed in the next chapter.

REFERENCES

1. Shang A, Tong Gan. Optimizing postoperative pain management in the ambulatory patient. *Drugs.* 2003;63(9):855–867.
2. Nicholas A, Oleski S. Osteopathic manipulative treatment for postoperative pain. *J Am Osteopath Assoc.* 2002;102(9):S5–S8.
3. Golden B. A multidisciplinary approach to nonpharmacologic pain management. *J Am Osteopath Assoc.* 2002;102(9):S1–S5.
4. Charlton E. The management of postoperative pain. *Update Anesth.* 1997;7:1–17.
5. Ilfeld B, Enneking FK. Continuous peripheral nerve blocks at home: A review. *Anesth Analg.* 2005;100:1822–1833.
6. Croll S, Shockey S. Advances in battlefield pain control. *ASA Newsl.* 2006;70(3): http://www.asahq.org/Newsletters/2006/03-06/croll03_06.html.
7. Beecher H. The powerful placebo. *JAMA.* 1955;159(17):1602–1606.

Alternative Pain Control

Cristin A. McMurray and Fred E. Shapiro

The traditional "Western view" of science and medicine involves the use of pharmacopoeias to control pain; however, there are other ways of understanding human behavior, medicine, and pain that deserve attention. As previously mentioned, the biopsychosocial model of pain suggests that other factors play into an individual's experience of pain. A significant amount of research has gone into mind–body therapies (MBTs) for the treatment of different types of pain, including postoperative pain. Often these techniques are used in conjunction with more traditional management in an attempt to improve patient comfort and reduce drug requirements. This is an area that has garnered much public and media attention in the last 20 years.

Several explanations have been offered for the success of MBTs (see Box 16.1).

Box 16.1 • Possible Reasons for the Success of Mind–Body Therapies

Attenuation of stress reactivity

Ability to cope more effectively with pain

Reinforcement of the patient's sense of control

Pain is frequently mediated by emotional and psychological factors; it is exacerbated by anxiety and a feeling of helplessness in the face of suffering. Researchers have hypothesized that MBTs may lessen the patient's state of sympathetic arousal and cause a "relaxation response" to facilitate greater control over stress reactivity. The state of hypoarousal induced by some MBTs may allow patients to develop a more detached stance toward their sensory experience of pain and reduce the emotional aspects of their pain. These MBT modalities also offer patients a means of asserting some control over their situation. Studies have shown that perceived self-efficacy is an important factor in pain tolerance. Although the actual physical experience of pain may not be altered by various MBTs, the patient's emotional and cognitive response may be lessened, allowing them to remain calmer, less anxious, and less distressed by the pain (1).

This chapter will explain some of the different MBT modalities, specifically those areas that are supported by evidence-based research and their use in the perioperative setting (see Box 16.2).

Box 16.2 • Mind–Body Therapies with Evidence-Based Research in the Perioperative Setting

Massage

Acupuncture

Music Therapy

Hypnosis

MASSAGE

Massage is the manipulation (touching, kneading) of soft tissues of the body for therapeutic purposes. Studies have shown that, when integrated in conjunction with opioid pain relief, massage is more effective than opioids alone in the treatment of acute postoperative pain.

Piotrowski et al. published an article in the Journal of the American College of Surgeons in 2003. They evaluated postoperative pain in 202 patients who underwent major operations and divided them into three groups of nursing interventions: massage (81), focused attention (66), or routine care (55). The interventions were performed twice daily for 10 minutes, beginning 24 hours after the operation through postoperative day 7. The patient population was fairly homogeneous, with more than 50% of the patients 60 years or older, 97% male, with the sternum as the most common incision site (77%). Routine care included administering medications, checking the patients' vital signs, checking the patients for comfort and safety, and performing wound care and dressing changes. In the focused attention group, in addition to the routine care described, dedicated time (10 minutes with the research nurse) was added to assess the effect of emotional support, independent of massage, on pain relief. No visitors were present and the door or curtain was closed to maintain privacy. The nurse sat close to the bed, facing the patient at a comfortable speaking distance in order to promote patient–nurse interaction. Either party could initiate a conversation or not; silence was acceptable.

The massage group, in addition to routine care, received a 10-minute effleurage back massage provided by the research nurse who had no prior formal training in massage. (Before the research study, each nurse was trained in this process by a 3- to 4-hour session with a certified massage therapist.) The back massage was given in the prone or lateral position, depending on where the wound was located. Moderate, firm massage strokes were used while the patient was urged to relax and advise the research nurse of any discomfort, or if he wanted to change positions, stop the massage, or change the technique.

During 82% of the focused attention group sessions and 71% of the massage sessions, participants discussed health care concerns. The two most common topics were pain and physical activities and limitations. Patients in the massage group believed that their treatment decreased discomfort 77% of the time; the focused attention group believed that the intervention decreased pain 64% of the time.

The greatest impact of this effect of focused attention or massage was during the first 72 hours postoperatively. When rating patient satisfaction, both experimental groups admitted that interventions improved their pain control, more so in the massage group. The most interesting finding of this study is that *massage significantly accelerated the rate of decline in pain unpleasantness*, as perceived by the patients. *This aspect of pain is often not elicited from patients but significantly impacts their recovery and experience of pain.* Based on the results of this study, it was recommended that massage might be a useful tool to palliate a patient's distress postoperatively (2).

In the office-based setting, massage may be a useful intervention to recommend to patients at home; many insurance plans are starting to reimburse patients for doctor-prescribed massage therapy sessions.

Acupuncture

Employed as a therapeutic intervention in traditional Chinese medicine, acupuncture is believed to work by maintaining and balancing the flow of Qi (chi) in the human body; Qi is a concept equated to "the vital energy," something that is difficult to translate into English. The concept of Qi is broad; it interconnects both living and inanimate objects in nature and the universe. Postulated by Chinese philosophy, it is a tangible force that allows energy transfer, movement, growth, and development to occur. To maintain physical and mental health, the flow of Qi must stay fluid and in balance, microscopically, as organ functions interact, and macroscopically, as individuals relate to their environment. An imbalance in the flow of Qi can manifest as disease. Individuals can influence the balance of Qi internally by analyzing the flow of Qi along defined pathways on the body surface in a set of channels called *meridians*. These meridians are all interconnected and connect to all body organs in a complex manner. Treatment occurs by first identifying the internal and external imbalances, then by inserting very fine needles into appropriate points along these meridians, helping to realign Qi flow in the body and restore internal homeostasis. Therefore, the basic premise of acupuncture, in simple terms, is that stimulation of one site on the body has an effect on another more distant site (3).

On a physiologic level, the sensation of pain begins with a stimulus, a surgical incision, for example. There are receptors in the body that respond to this stimulus and, through specific nerve fibers, convey this information to the spinal cord. Here, they interconnect with additional nerve fibers to transfer this message to higher areas in the brain, namely the thalamus, hypothalamus, and cerebral cortex, where the perception of pain occurs. Immediately, this stimulus initiates a behavioral response on the part of the patient, for example, "ouch!" This, in turn, activates another area in the brain that stimulates production of endogenous opioidlike substances (endorphins, dynorphins, enkephalins) that travel back down to the spinal cord, through the descending inhibitory pathway, in order to modulate or inhibit this nociceptive information. *Acupuncture has been shown to influence pain perception by modulating the activity at the descending inhibitory pathway and subsequently decreasing the requirement of pain medications, for example, opioids.* These results were reiterated in a study that determined that preoperative insertion of acupuncture needles at traditional acupuncture points decreased supplemental morphine consumption by 50% (4). Obviously, in order to use acupuncture in the office setting, one would need additional training, or have a certified acupuncturist on staff. Although this may seem a bit extreme, there is interest in acupuncture among patients as well as some physicians. Many hospitals are starting to incorporate acupuncturists into their clinical practice. An overall patient cost–benefit analysis might be the next step for research.

Music Therapy

Although most people enjoy music in the operating room (OR), some music may help modulate patients' responses to pain postoperatively. *Soothing music or music with relaxation suggestions in the postoperative period can increase the benefit of medication, decrease the response to stress, and increase satisfaction with preoperative care.* Nillson et al. published an interesting article, which looked at whether the benefits of music or music in combination with therapeutic suggestions could improve the postoperative recovery in ambulatory surgery.

In this study, 182 patients were randomly divided into three groups: (a) listening to music, (b) music in combination with therapeutic suggestions, or (c) a blank tape in the immediate postoperative period. The method of anesthesia, surgical technique, and postoperative pain medication were all standardized, and the music was soft classical compositions. The relaxing and encouraging suggestions were recorded by a male voice with an extensive background in hypnotherapy. *The taped voice suggested a feeling of relaxation, security, rapid healing, return to normal appetite, quick recovery, absence of pain and nausea, together with encouragement of comfort.* The blank tape was simply that, a blank tape, that is, silence. All tape players were set at the same level to permit conversation between the patient, nurse, and physicians in the postanesthesia care unit (PACU). Pain medication requirements, nausea, fatigue, anxiety, headache, well-being, urinary problems, heart rate, and oxygen saturation were evaluated in the PACU as outcome variables. Each group had ~ 60 patients, the average age was 50 years, male:female ratio was 40:20. The procedures were inguinal hernia repairs and varicose vein stripping, with an average duration of surgery of approximately 40 minutes and average duration of anesthesia of approximately 65 minutes. Patients in both the music alone and music with therapeutic suggestion groups complained of less pain intensity postoperatively; however, there was no significant difference in the amount of pain medication requirement between the groups. There was no difference in the heart rate, anxiety, nausea, well-being, fatigue, urinary problems, and headache on the day of surgery and the first postoperative day. All patients remembered that they were listening to music or music in combination with therapeutic suggestions.

In the PACU, the noise is mainly generated from the staff or equipment. It is thought that perhaps the beneficial effects were due to the music acting simply as a distracter from the environmental noise in the PACU rather than due to the behavioral intervention.

It was the author's opinion that taped music, with or without therapeutic suggestions, is an inexpensive, noninvasive, nonpharmacologic technique that should be offered to patients because of its beneficial effects in decreasing pain and anxiety. Although they may not have achieved statistically significant differences in vital signs, patients' perceptions of pain were improved (5).

Playing a patient's favorite music CD or iPOD in the perioperative setting maximizes the soothing effect of music.

Hypnosis

Hypnosis has been shown to have beneficial effects in the postoperative setting. What does hypnosis entail in the perioperative arena? In a clinical setting, it is established by an "induction" procedure, in which the hypnotist guides the patient through peaceful and relaxing imagery with the goal of making her feel more relaxed, distracted from aversive stimuli, and open to therapeutic suggestions. The induction phase is followed by an application phase, in which the hypnotist makes suggestions to the patient; these suggestions may include changes in sensory or cognitive processes, physiology (e.g., heart rate) or behavior. Examples include *suggestions for reduced pain, reduced stress, increased vitality, and an increased sense of personal efficacy*. During hypnotic induction, verbal instructions may stimulate physical changes, whereas a change in mental state can produce alterations in the physical state. This same phenomenon can be accomplished by the pharmacologic alterations of drugs. On the basis of this reasoning, one can appreciate how the use of hypnosis can be integrated as a nonpharmacologic adjunct in the approach to surgical patients. The effects can also be achieved with a tape-recorded presentation of hypnosis interventions. After recovery from hypnosedation, patients report a feeling of well-being and a high degree of satisfaction.

Faymonville's study looked at 337 patients having monitored anesthesia care (MAC) for various plastic surgery procedures and divided them into three groups. The first group received alfentanil and midazolam. The second group received the same medications and, in addition, achieved a hypnotic "trance" level and relaxation. The third group received the same medications, and hypnosis was induced, without achieving a full "trance level." The groups with hypnosis and relaxation had less anxiety intraoperatively, less pain intra- and postoperatively, and the drug requirements of narcotic and anxiolytic were decreased; patients also experienced a decrease in the incidence of postoperative nausea and vomiting (PONV). Overall, greater patient satisfaction was obtained with the anesthetic procedure and greater surgical comfort was reported in the hypnosis group (6).

Another randomized controlled study looked at the effects of hypnosis on postsurgical wound healing. Although the study size was small (18 women undergoing reduction mammoplasty), the results were suggestive. The patients were divided into three groups—six women attended 8 half-hour weekly hypnosis sessions starting 2 weeks preoperatively and continuing 6 weeks after the surgery, six women attended "supportive attention" sessions for the same time periods as the hypnosis sessions, and six control women had regular care and postoperative visits. The women who had hypnosis were judged to have significantly greater wound healing over time than the other two groups by surgeons blinded to group identities viewing photographs at 1 and 7 weeks postoperatively. Additionally, the women in the hypnosis group had lower self-reported scores for pain, albeit not statistically significant, but notable (7).

The suggestion of pleasant experiences is more effective in producing pain relief than the suggestion of declining pain. A hypnotic trance results in a state of dissociation, which may allow for the separation of the pain sensation from the subjective experience of feeling pain. Furthermore, it has been noted that hypnosis-induced pain relief persists after the completion of surgery and the cessation of hypnosis. It is theorized that intraoperative hypnosis may produce pre-emptive analgesia. If this could be confirmed, then the implication is that psychological manipulation can induce biochemical changes, a very exciting concept. This same mechanism may explain the relief of anxiety. *Hypnosis allows* for the transition from a passive suffering state to one that is active and independent. This permits *a change in the subjective experience and perception of the patient* (Table 16.1).

Table 16.1. Evidence-based research on mind–body therapies

Modalities	Study	Clinically Relevant Conclusions
Massage	Piotrowski, 2003. J Am Coll Surg	"Focused attention" and massage groups reported interventions improved pain control, especially first 72 h postoperatively; decrease in "pain unpleasantness"
Acupuncture	Kotani et al., 2001. Anethesiology; Audette and Ryan, 2004. Phys Med Rehabil Clin N Am, Pain Principles and Practice of Acupuncture	Decrease in supplemental morphine consumption postoperatively
Music	Nilsson et al., 2003. Acta Anesthesiol Scand	Patients complained of less pain intensity postoperatively; no significant decrease in pain medications or other physiologic variables
Hypnosis	Faymonville et al., 1995. Reg Anesth	Hypnosis and relaxation groups had less perioperative anxiety, pain, and drug requirements; also less PONV; better patient satisfaction and surgical comfort
	Ginandes et al, 2003. Am J Clin Hypn	Hypnosis patients judged to have greater wound healing by blinded surgeons postoperatively

PONV, postoperative nausea and vomiting.

CONCLUSIONS

Despite practitioners' mixed feelings about complementary and alternative medicine (CAM) or MBT, savvy patients are interested in these treatments, and some studies suggest that they may have an important role to play in helping treat perioperative pain in the office-based setting. Certainly, some interventions, such as calming music in the PACU, are easy and inexpensive means that can be adapted into clinical practice quite readily. However, because the treatment of postoperative pain can be better, it seems reasonable to investigate alternate means of therapy, which can work together with more traditional medications, without adding side effects.

REFERENCES

1. Astin J. Mind-body therapies for the management of pain. *Clin J Pain*. 2004; 20(1):27–32.
2. Piotrowski M. Massage as adjuvant therapy in the management of acute postoperative pain: A preliminary study in men. *J Am Coll Surg*. 2003;197(6): 1037–1046.
3. Audette J, Ryan A. The role of acupuncture in pain management. *Phys Med Rehabil Clin N Am*. 2004;15(4):749–772.
4. Kotani N, Hasimoto H, Sato Y, et al. Preoperative intradermal acupuncture reduces postoperative pain, nausea and vomiting, analgesic requirement and sympathoadrenal responses. *Anesthesiology*. 2001;95(2):349–356.
5. Nilsson U, Rawal N, Enqvist B, et al. Analgesia following music and therapeutic suggestions in the PACU in ambulatory surgery; a randomized controlled trial. *Acta Anaesthesiol Scand*. 2003;47(3):278–283.
6. Faymonville ME, Fissette J, Mambourg PH, et al. Hypnosis as adjunct therapy in conscious sedation for plastic surgery. *Reg Anesth*. 1995;20(2):145–151.
7. Ginandes C, Brooks P, Sando W, et al. Can medical hypnosis accelerate post-surgical wound healing? results of a clinical trial. *Am J Clin Hypn*. 2003;45: 333–351.

Postanesthesia Care Unit—Recovery and Discharge

Pankaj K. Sikka

The creation of modern postanesthesia care units (PACU) has significantly reduced the morbidity and mortality associated with anesthesia and surgery. In the office-based setting, over the last 10 years, we have seen a dramatic increase in the number of procedures, the complexity of the procedures, and the American Society of Anesthesiology (ASA) status of the patients (1). More complex surgical procedures for durations up to 6 hours are now being performed on sicker patients.

Potentially life-threatening complications usually occur in the first few hours after anesthesia or surgery. This is supported by the results of the ASA Closed Claim Analysis regarding office-based claims; the most common mechanism of injury was due to respiratory events in the postoperative period (2,3). Furthermore, these events were deemed preventable by the addition of pulse oximetry in the recovery period (4,5). Therefore, all patients regardless of the type of anesthesia (i.e., general, regional, or monitored anesthesia care [MAC]) upon completion of surgery should be admitted to the PACU. Once the effects of anesthesia begin to wear off, patients may then be transferred out of the PACU or discharged home.

POSTANESTHESIA CARE UNIT—DESIGN AND EQUIPMENT

The PACU should be located as near to the ORs as possible, if need arises to take the patient back there (see Box 17.1). Usually, patients are observed in the PACU in open designated areas. Few spaces are designated "enclosed" areas to observe patients needing isolation. Each PACU space should be well lighted, easily accessible, and should have enough space available for equipment such as a ventilator or an x-ray machine. In addition, outlets for oxygen and suction should be available.

Box 17.1 • Design

- Close proximity to the operating room (OR)
- Open designated area
- Well lighted
- Easily accessible
- Allow room for equipment
- Electrical outlets

Standard equipment for monitoring a PACU patient should include a pulse oximeter, electrocardiograph (ECG) and an automated blood pressure cuff (see Box 17.2). Transducers for monitoring arterial, central, and pulmonary artery pressures should be available (see Box 17.3). Temperature is usually determined by the PACU nurse on the patient's admission to the PACU. If hypothermic, the patient can be warmed using a forced air–warming device.

Box 17.2 • Standard Equipment

- Oxygen
- Suction
- Pulse oximeter
- Electrocardiogram
- Blood pressure monitor
- Temperature monitor

Box 17.3 • Emergency Equipment

- Airway = oral/nasal airways, oxygen cannulae
- Breathing = face masks, endotracheal tubes, laryngoscopes, and laryngeal mask airways (LMAs)
- Circulation = intravenous catheters and fluids
- Drugs = emergency cart containing all life support equipment

---

PATIENT TRANSPORT TO AND FROM THE POSTANESTHESIA CARE UNIT

Once the surgery is completed, the patient is transferred to a stretcher to be taken to the PACU. Oxygen supplementation should be available and given to the patient through nasal cannula/face mask connected to an appropriately full oxygen tank. Monitors with the ability to monitor pulse oximetry, ECG, and blood pressure should be available, if needed. On reaching the PACU, oxygen supplementation is switched to a wall source and the patient is appropriately monitored (pulse oximetry, ECG, and blood pressure). Finally, a report is given to the PACU nurse with details about the anesthesia given and the surgery performed.

MANAGEMENT TEAM

Fully trained nurses should be available to take care of the patients in the PACU. The PACU should be under the direct medical direction of the anesthesiologist, if possible. The anesthesiologist usually manages analgesia, pulmonary, or cardiac complications, whereas the surgeon usually manages complications directly related to the procedure. A PACU nurse is assigned to take care of not more than two patients at any given time. Depending on the complexity of the surgery and the severity of the illness of the patient, a PACU can be divided into a regular PACU area, a secondary recovery area (SRA) mainly for ambulatory surgical patients, and an extended observation unit (EOU) for patients needing >4 to 6 hours to be discharged from the PACU.

Although these designations are ideal for an ambulatory center, in the office-based setting, the areas might not be as well defined. However, the principle and premise should remain the same.

DISCHARGE CRITERIA FROM THE POSTANESTHESIA CARE UNIT

Discharge from the PACU usually depends on meeting all or most of the criteria mentioned in Box 17.4 and Table 17.1. The anesthesiology department and the hospital administration usually set these criteria. An anesthesiologist is usually assigned to sign the patient out of the PACU. Several discharge/postanesthesia recovery scores are available (e.g., Aldrete score (6,7) and Postanesthesia Discharge Scoring [PADS] System (8)) which can be used by individual hospitals to establish discharge criteria (see Table 17.2).

Table 17.1.   Criteria for discharge from the postanesthesia care unit

	Extended Criteria
Central nervous system	Awake, alert, oriented, moves all extremities
Airway and breathing	Can take deep breaths, color pink, and oxygen saturation >92% on room air
Circulatory	Stable vital signs
Renal	Ability to void urine
Gastrointestinal	Absence of severe nausea/vomiting, able to tolerate fluids
Pain	Control of significant pain
Regional anesthesia	Resolution of a spinal/epidural block
Temperature	Normothermia
Major surgical complications	Absent
Home discharge	Ride available

Box 17.4 • Minimum Criteria

- Hemodynamically stable
- Adequate pain control
- No nausea or vomiting

Once the patient meets the discharge criteria (a score of at least 10), the patient is discharged from the PACU and should be accompanied by a designated person (family or friend) who is responsible for safe transport to home. Patients who need to be transported for further evaluation should have oxygen supplementation and appropriate monitors, as needed.

The decision to "bypass" the PACU (a score of at least 12), if at all, should be made in conference by the anesthesiologist and the surgeon. This should depend on the procedure, the patient's comorbidities, any intraoperative events, and the amount of anesthesia administered (MAC/general anesthesia [GA]) (see Table 17.3). Along with the growing number and complexity of patients and cases, we cannot emphasize enough how important it is that all office-based facilities have the mechanism immediately available to emergently transport the patient to a nearby tertiary care hospital, if needed.

RESUMPTION OF NORMAL ACTIVITIES FOR AMBULATORY PATIENTS

Oral Intake

Awake, alert, non-nauseated patients can be offered ice-chips, water, or clear juice. If these are tolerated well, then crackers, gelatin, or even a light sandwich may be offered. The type of surgery may, however, limit the oral intake in some patients. Judgment of whether mandatory fluid consumption is required before discharge should be made on an individual basis.

Physical Activities

It is important that patients discharged from the PACU should have a ride available to their destination (home/nursing facility). The patients may be drowsy and may need a day or two to get their system rid of the anesthetic medication to operate machinery. Resumption of physical activities also depends on the type of surgery, location of the incision, and adequate pain control.

Table 17.2. Modified Aldrete scoring system

Level of Consciousness	Score
Awake	2
Arousable	1
Minimally (tactile) responsive	0
Physical activity	
Moves all extremities	2
Some weakness	1
Unable to move extremities	0
Hemodynamic stability	
MABP <15% off baseline	2
MABP 15%–30% off baseline	1
MABP >30% off baseline	0
Respiration	
Can take deep breaths	2
Tachypnea with good cough	1
Dyspneic with weak cough	0
Oxygen saturation	
>90% room air	2
Requires supplemental oxygen	1
<90% with oxygen	0
Postoperative pain	
None or mild	2
Moderate	1
Severe	0
Nausea/vomiting	
None or mild nausea	2
Transient vomiting	1
Moderate to severe nausea/vomiting	0
Total score	14

MABP, mean arterial blood pressure.

POSTANESTHESIA CARE UNIT PROBLEMS

There are six major problems that cause time-to-discharge delays and unanticipated hospital admissions (see Box 17.5).

Box 17.5

- Delayed emergence from anesthesia
- Airway obstruction
- Pain
- Nausea/vomiting
- Urinary retention
- Hypothermia and shivering

Table 17.3.   Strategies for quicker emergence from anesthesia and shorter postanesthesia care unit stay length

Sedation	Midazolam, dexmedetomidine
Pain	Fentanyl, dexmedetomidine
Intravenous induction agent	Propofol
Inhalational agent for general anesthesia	Desflurane or sevoflurane
Anesthesia technique	Laryngeal mask airway (LMA) vs. endotracheal intubation, appropriate use of regional anesthesia techniques
Nausea prevention	Metoclopramide, ondansetron, and/or dexamethasone
Temperature control—normothermia	Forced air–warming device, humidifier
Hydration	Adequate (usually <1 L in healthy patients undergoing minor surgery)

Delayed Emergence from Anesthesia

The primary cause of delayed emergence from GA is hypoventilation. Therefore, using an inhalational agent with a fast on and off time (low blood gas solubility) such as desflurane or sevoflurane would reduce the emergence time from anesthesia, and hence the length of the PACU stay. Advanced age with a decreased ability to metabolize drugs and the presence of renal or hepatic disease could also significantly delay emergence from anesthesia.

Using drugs with a shorter elimination half-life is very important to facilitate emergence from anesthesia. Examples of these drugs include midazolam (a benzodiazepine, used instead of Valium), fentanyl (an opioid, used instead of morphine), vecuronium (a neuromuscular relaxing agent, used instead of pancuronium), dexmedetomidine (an α_2 agonist) used for its sedative, analgesic, cardiorespiratory stability and MAC-sparing effects. Opioid overdose and side effects (nausea, vomiting, pruritus, and urinary retention) may be treated with an antagonist naloxone (1–5 μg/kg). Benzodiazepine overdose may be treated with flumazenil (200 μg, every 3 minutes till effect, total of 3 mg).

Airway Obstruction

A patient being brought to the PACU may have labored breathing due to the tongue falling back and obstructing the pharynx ("ball-valve effect"). A simple jaw-thrust maneuver and providing supplemental oxygen usually relieves the airway obstruction. However, it should be remembered that airway obstruction might also be due to excessive secretions, blood in the airway (ENT surgery), airway edema and laryngospasm.

Laryngospasm (stimulation of the superior laryngeal nerve), glottic edema/postextubation stridor and bronchospasm are life threatening and should be treated emergently (see Boxes 17.6, 17.7 and 17.8).

Box 17.6 • Treatment of Laryngospasm

- 100% oxygen
- Positive airway pressure
- Succinylcholine 20–40 mg IV

Box 17.7 • Treatment of Glottic Edema

- 100% oxygen
- Glucocorticoids
- Racemic epinephrine (nebulized)

Box 17.8 • Treatment of Bronchospasm

- β_2 Agonists (nebulized albuterol 0.2–0.3 mL in 2–3 mL normal saline); if refractory, add
- Epinephrine (0.3 mL, 1:1,000)

Pain

Opioids remain the cornerstone in managing postoperative pain. Commonly used opioids include fentanyl, morphine, and hydromorphone. These are usually administered intravenously or epidurally if the patient has an epidural catheter. A newer opiate drug is remifentanil (9) with a quick onset and offset time (IV infusion of 0.1–0.5 μg/kg/min). Patients should be closely watched for any respiratory depressive effects of the opioids. Patients with severe pain may be started on a patient-controlled analgesia (PCA) to better manage the pain.

Nonopioid drugs used for managing pain usually include ketorolac, ketamine in small doses (usually as an adjuvant), or even intravenously acetaminophen (Tylenol, in Europe). Oral analgesics include acetaminophen alone or in combination with propoxyphene napsylate (Darvocet), oxycodone (Percocet), codeine and hydrocodone (Vicodin). For recommended dosing, refer to Chapter 15.

Nausea and/or Vomiting

Nausea and vomiting are commonly seen in the PACU after administration of anesthesia (10). Causes may include use of nitrous oxide, inhalational agent, opioids (GA), hypotension from a regional anesthesia or hypovolemia and the type of surgery (laparoscopic or gynecology surgery) (see Box 17.9).

Box 17.9 • Common Causes of Nausea/Vomiting

- Nitrous oxide
- Inhalation agent
- Opioids
- Type of surgery (laparoscopic, gynecologic, strabismus-eye, inguinal hernia)

See Box 17.10 for the prevention and treatment of nausea. Other drugs available are a transdermal scopolamine patch and antihistaminics such as promethazine and diphenhydramine. Patients with full stomach/prone to pulmonary aspiration (hiatal hernia, obesity, pregnancy) may benefit from pre-emptive treatment with antiemetic agents.

Box 17.10 • Prevention/Treatment of Nausea

- Drugs (metoclopramide, ondansetron, droperidol, dexamethasone)
- Adequate hydration
- Pain control

Urinary Retention

This is common after a regional anesthetic but can also occur after GA (11). Urinary retention may cause patient agitation and restlessness. Evacuation of the bladder by a single catheter insertion or a Foley's catheter may be required. Hypoxemia should also be ruled out in an agitated and restless patient.

Hypothermia and Shivering

Most general anesthetic agents cause vasodilatation, which causes heat loss leading to hypothermia (12). The proposed physiologic mechanism for this is heat dissipation between the "core and peripheral compartments" of the body. The most common mechanism (85%) of heat loss is due to radiation. Other causes of hypothermia include exposure of a large wound, cold intravenous fluids, and a low OR temperature. Shivering may result because of the hypothermia so as to increase heat production and the body temperature. Although shivering increases the body temperature, it also causes increased oxygen consumption, carbon dioxide production and cardiac output, which may be detrimental to patients with existing cardiac or pulmonary diseases (see Box 17.11).

Box 17.11 • Methods Used to Attenuate/Prevent Hypothermia

- Forced air–warming device
- Warming intravenous fluids
- Using a humidifier within the breathing circuit
- Raising the ambient room temperature
- Meperidine, 12.5–25 mg IV, can be used to stop shivering

CIRCULATORY PROBLEMS

Hypertension

Postoperative hypertension may occur because of the presence of pain, hypoxia, or bladder distension (see Box 17.12) (13). Severe hypertension may lead to myocardial ischemia or cerebral bleeding. Every effort should be made to keep the blood pressure within 20% to 30% of the patient's baseline. Treatment of postoperative hypertension includes the treatment of surgical pain with narcotics, intravenous β-adrenergic blockers (labetalol, esmolol, metoprolol), hydralazine, or more acutely with nitroglycerin or nitroprusside (see Box 17.13).

Box 17.12 • Etiology

- Hypoxia
- Pain
- Bladder distension

Box 17.13 • Treatment

IV administration of the following:
- Narcotics
- βBlockers
- Hydralazine
- Nitroglycerine
- Nitroprusside

Hypotension

The most common cause of hypotension in the PACU is hypovolemia (see Box 17.14). This is usually due to an inadequate replacement of fluid/blood lost by the patient, intraoperatively. Other causes of hypotension include sepsis, allergic drug reactions, and impaired cardiac function. Hypotension can be treated by identifying the cause, administration of fluid/blood, treatment of sepsis, treatment of allergic reactions (anaphylaxis—epinephrine) or treatment of myocardial ischemia (see Box 17.15).

Box 17.14 • Etiology

- Hypovolemia
- Sepsis
- Allergic reaction
- Cardiac dysfunction

Box 17.15 • Treatment: Identify the Cause and Treat Accordingly

- Fluid/blood (hypovolemia)
- Antibiotics (sepsis)
- Diphenhydramine, epinephrine (allergic reaction)
- Oxygen, nitrates, ECG (myocardial ischemia)

Cardiac Arrhythmias

A patient recovering from anesthesia and surgery is prone to develop arrhythmias (see Box 17.16).

Box 17.16 • Etiology

- Anesthetic drugs
- Hypoxemia
- Hypercarbia
- Pain
- Sympathetic overactivity
- Metabolic acidosis
- Metabolic abnormalities

Appropriate drugs should be available to treat these arrhythmias and also the presence of a nearby defibrillator (see Box 17.17 and Appendices 7–11).

Box 17.17 • Common Arrhythmias

- Bradycardia
- Tachycardia
- Premature atrial and ventricular ectopic beats
- Atrial flutter/fibrillation
- Ventricular tachycardia

REFERENCES

1. Coyle TT, Helfrick JF, Gonzalez ML, et al. Office-based ambulatory anesthesia: Factors that influence patient satisfaction or dissatisfaction with deep sedation/general anesthesia. *J Oral Maxillofac Surg*. 2005;63:163–172.
2. Chung F, Mezei G. Adverse outcomes in ambulatory anesthesia. *Can J Anaesth*. 1999;46(5):R18–R26.
3. Kallar SK, Jones GW. Postoperative complications. In: White PF, ed. *Outpatient anesthesia*. New York: Churchill Livingstone; 1990:397–415.
4. Chung F, Un V, Su J. Postoperative symptoms 24 hours after ambulatory anaesthesia. *Can J Anaesth*. 1996;43(11):1121–1127.
5. Warner MA, Shields SE, Chute CG. Major morbidity and mortality within 1 month of ambulatory surgery and anesthesia. *JAMA*. 1993;270(12): 1437–1441.
6. Aldrete JA, Kroulik D. A postanesthetic recovery score. *Anesth Analg*. 1970;49:924–934.
7. White PF, Song D. New criteria for fast-tracking after outpatient anesthesia: A comparison with the modified Aldrete's scoring system. *Anesth Analg*. 1999;88:1069–1072.
8. Kallar SK, Chung F. Practical application of postanesthetic discharge scoring system-PADSS. *Anesthesiology*. 1992;77:A12.
9. Roscow C. Remifentanil: A unique opioid analgesic. *Anesthesiology*. 1993;79: 875–876.
10. Watcha MF, White PF. Postoperative nausea and vomiting: Its etiology, treatment and prevention. *Anesthesiology*. 1992;77:162–184.
11. Bridenbaugh LD. Regional anaesthesia for outpatient surgery-a summary of 12 years experience. *Can Anaesth Soc J*. 1983;30:548–552.
12. Slotman GJ, Jed EH. Adverse effects of hypothermia in postoperative patients. *Am J Surg*. 1985;149:495–501.
13. Gal TJ, Cooperman LH. Hypertension in the immediate postoperative period. *Br J Anaesth*. 1975;40:70–74.

Appendix 1

GUIDELINES FOR AMBULATORY ANESTHESIA AND SURGERY (APPROVED BY HOUSE OF DELEGATES ON OCTOBER 11, 1973, AND LAST AFFIRMED ON OCTOBER 15, 2003)

The American Society of Anesthesiologists (ASA) endorses and supports the concept of ambulatory anesthesia and surgery. ASA encourages the anesthesiologist to play a leadership role as the perioperative physician in all hospitals, ambulatory surgical facilities and office-based settings.

These guidelines apply to all care involving anesthesiology personnel administering ambulatory anesthesia in all settings. These are minimal guidelines, which may be exceeded at any time based on the judgment of the involved anesthesia personnel. These guidelines encourage high quality patient care, but observing them cannot guarantee any specific patient outcome. These guidelines are subject to periodic revision, as warranted by the evolution of technology and practice.

I. ASA standards, guidelines and policies should be adhered to in all settings except where they are not applicable to outpatient care.

II. A licensed physician should be in attendance in the facility, or in the case of overnight care, immediately available by telephone, at all times during patient treatment and recovery and until the patients are medically discharged.

III. The facility must be established, constructed, equipped, and operated in accordance with applicable local, state, and federal laws and regulations. At a minimum, all settings should have a reliable source of oxygen, suction, resuscitation equipment, and emergency drugs. (Specific reference is made to the ASA *"Guidelines for Nonoperating Room Anesthetizing Locations."*)

IV. Staff should be adequate to meet patient and facility needs for all procedures performed in the setting, and should consist of the following:

    A. Professional staff

        1. Physicians and other practitioners who hold a valid license or certificate are duly qualified.

        2. Nurses who are duly licensed and qualified.

    B. Administrative staff

    C. Housekeeping and maintenance staff

V. Physicians providing medical care in the facility should assume responsibility for credentials review, delineation of privileges, quality assurance, and peer review.

VI. Qualified personnel and equipment should be on hand to manage emergencies. There should be established policies and procedures to respond to emergencies and unanticipated patient transfer to an acute care facility.

VII. Minimal patient care should include the following:

    A. Preoperative instructions and preparation.

    B. An appropriate preanesthesia evaluation and examination by an anesthesiologist, before anesthesia and surgery. In the event that nonphysician personnel are utilized in the process, the anesthesiologist must verify the information and repeat and record essential key elements of the evaluation.

    C. Preoperative studies and consultations as medically indicated.

    D. An anesthesia plan developed by an anesthesiologist and discussed with and accepted by the patient.

    E. Administration of anesthesia by anesthesiologists, other qualified physicians or nonphysician anesthesia personnel medically directed by an anesthesiologist.

    F. Discharge of the patient is a physician responsibility.

G. Patients who receive other than unsupplemented local anesthesia must be discharged with a responsible adult.
H. Written postoperative and follow-up care instructions.
I. Accurate, confidential, and current medical records.

GUIDELINES FOR NONOPERATING ROOM ANESTHETIZING LOCATIONS (APPROVED BY HOUSE OF DELEGATES ON OCTOBER 19, 1994, AND LAST AMENDED ON OCTOBER 15, 2003)

These guidelines apply to all anesthesia care involving anesthesiology personnel for procedures intended to be performed in locations outside an operating room. These are minimal guidelines, which may be exceeded at any time based on the judgment of the involved anesthesia personnel. These guidelines encourage quality patient care but observing them cannot guarantee any specific patient outcome. These guidelines are subject to revision from time to time, as warranted by the evolution of technology and practice. ASA standards, guidelines and policies should be adhered to in all nonoperating room settings except where they are not applicable to the individual patient or care setting.

1. There should be in each location a reliable source of oxygen adequate for the length of the procedure. There should also be a backup supply. Before administering any anesthetic, the anesthesiologist should consider the capabilities, limitations, and accessibility of both the primary and backup oxygen sources. Oxygen piped from a central source, meeting applicable codes, is strongly encouraged. The backup system should include the equivalent of at least a full E cylinder.
2. There should be in each location an adequate and reliable source of suction. Suction apparatus that meets operating room standards is strongly encouraged.
3. In any location in which inhalation anesthetics are administered, there should be an adequate and reliable system for scavenging waste anesthetic gases.
4. There should be in each location: (a) a self-inflating hand resuscitator bag capable of administering at least 90% oxygen as a means to deliver positive pressure ventilation; (b) adequate anesthesia drugs, supplies and equipment for the intended anesthesia care; and (c) adequate monitoring equipment to allow adherence to the "Standards for Basic Anesthetic Monitoring." In any location in which inhalation anesthesia is to be administered, there should be an anesthesia machine equivalent in function to that employed in operating rooms and maintained to current operating room standards.
5. There should be in each location, sufficient electrical outlets to satisfy anesthesia machine and monitoring equipment requirements, including clearly labeled outlets connected to an emergency power supply. In any anesthetizing location determined by the health care facility to be a "wet location" (e.g., for cystoscopy or arthroscopy or a birthing room in labor and delivery), either isolated electric power or electric circuits with ground fault circuit interrupters should be provided.[1]
6. There should be in each location, provision for adequate illumination of the patient, anesthesia machine (when present) and monitoring equipment. In addition, a form of battery-powered illumination other than a laryngoscope should be immediately available.
7. There should be in each location, sufficient space to accommodate necessary equipment and personnel and to allow expeditious access to the patient, anesthesia machine (when present) and monitoring equipment.

[1]See National Fire Protection Association. *Health Care Facilities Code* 99: Quincy, MA: NFPA; 1993.

8. There should be immediately available in each location, an emergency cart with a defibrillator, emergency drugs, and other equipment adequate to provide cardiopulmonary resuscitation.
9. There should be in each location adequate staff trained to support the anesthesiologist. There should be immediately available in each location, a reliable means of two-way communication to request assistance.
10. For each location, all applicable building and safety codes and facility standards, where they exist, should be observed.
11. Appropriate postanesthesia management should be provided (see Standards for Postanesthesia Care). In addition to the anesthesiologist, adequate numbers of trained staff and appropriate equipment should be available to safely transport the patient to a postanesthesia care unit.

GUIDELINES FOR OFFICE-BASED ANESTHESIA (APPROVED BY ASA HOUSE OF DELEGATES ON OCTOBER 13, 1999, AND LAST AFFIRMED ON OCTOBER 27, 2004)

These guidelines are intended to assist ASA members who are considering the practice of ambulatory anesthesia in the office setting: office-based anesthesia (OBA). These recommendations focus on quality anesthesia care and patient safety in the office. These are minimal guidelines and may be exceeded at any time based on the judgment of the involved anesthesia personnel. Compliance with these guidelines cannot guarantee any specific outcome. These guidelines are subject to periodic revision as warranted by the evolution of federal, state, and local laws as well as technology and practice.

ASA recognizes the unique needs of this growing practice and the increased requests for ASA members to provide OBA for health care practitioners[2] who have developed their own office operatories. Since OBA is a subset of ambulatory anesthesia, the ASA "Guidelines for Ambulatory Anesthesia and Surgery" should be followed in the office setting as well as all other ASA standards and guidelines that are applicable.

There are special problems that ASA members must recognize when administering anesthesia in the office setting. Compared with acute care hospitals and licensed ambulatory surgical facilities, office operatories currently have little or no regulation, oversight, or control by federal, state, or local laws. Therefore, ASA members must satisfactorily investigate areas taken for granted in the hospital or ambulatory surgical facility such as governance, organization, construction, and equipment, as well as policies and procedures, including fire, safety, drugs, emergencies, staffing, training, and unanticipated patient transfers.

ASA members should be confident that the following issues are addressed in an office setting to provide patient safety and to reduce risk and liability to the anesthesiologist.

ADMINISTRATION AND FACILITY
Quality of Care
- The facility should have a medical director or governing body that establishes policy and is responsible for the activities of the facility and its staff. The medical director or governing body is responsible for ensuring that facilities and personnel are adequate and appropriate for the type of procedures performed.
- Policies and procedures should be written for the orderly conduct of the facility and reviewed on an annual basis.
- The medical director or governing body should ensure that all applicable local, state and federal regulations are observed.
- All health care practitioners[2] and nurses should hold a valid license or certificate to perform their assigned duties.

[2]Defined herein as physicians, dentists, and podiatrists.

- All operating room personnel who provide clinical care in the office should be qualified to perform services commensurate with appropriate levels of education, training, and experience.
- The anesthesiologist should participate in ongoing continuous quality improvement and risk management activities.
- The medical director or governing body should recognize the basic human rights of its patients, and a written document that describes this policy should be available for patients to review.

Facility and Safety

- Facilities should comply with all applicable federal, state, and local laws, codes and regulations pertaining to fire prevention, building construction, and occupancy, accommodations for the disabled, occupational safety and health, and disposal of medical waste and hazardous waste.
- Policies and procedures should comply with laws and regulations pertaining to controlled drug supply, storage, and administration.

Clinical Care

Patient and Procedure Selection

- The anesthesiologist should be satisfied that the procedure to be undertaken is within the scope of practice of the health care practitioners and the capabilities of the facility.
- The procedure should be of a duration and degree of complexity that will permit the patient to recover and be discharged from the facility.
- Patients who by reason of pre-existing medical or other conditions may be at undue risk for complications should be referred to an appropriate facility for performance of the procedure and the administration of anesthesia.

Perioperative Care

- The anesthesiologist should adhere to the "Basic Standards for Preanesthesia Care," "Standards for Basic Anesthetic Monitoring," "Standards for Postanesthesia Care," and "Guidelines for Ambulatory Anesthesia and Surgery" as currently promulgated by the ASA.
- The anesthesiologist should be physically present during the intraoperative period and immediately available until the patient has been discharged from anesthesia care.
- Discharge of the patient is a physician responsibility. This decision should be documented in the medical record.
- Personnel with training in advanced resuscitative techniques (e.g., advanced cardiac life support [ACLS], pediatric advanced life support [PALS]) should be immediately available until all patients are discharged home.

Monitoring and Equipment

- At a minimum, all facilities should have a reliable source of oxygen, suction, resuscitation equipment, and emergency drugs. Specific reference is made to the ASA "Guidelines for Nonoperating Room Anesthetizing Locations."
- There should be sufficient space to accommodate all necessary equipment and personnel and to allow for expeditious access to the patient, anesthesia machine (when present), and all monitoring equipment.
- All equipment should be maintained, tested, and inspected according to the manufacturer's specifications.
- Backup power sufficient to ensure patient protection in the event of an emergency should be available.
- In any location in which anesthesia is administered, there should be appropriate anesthesia apparatus and equipment which allow monitoring consistent with ASA "Standards for Basic Anesthetic Monitoring" and

documentation of regular preventive maintenance as recommended by the manufacturer.

- In an office where anesthesia services are to be provided to infants and children, the required equipment, medication and resuscitative capabilities should be appropriately sized for a pediatric population.

Emergencies and Transfers

- All facility personnel should be appropriately trained in and regularly review the facility's written emergency protocols.
- There should be written protocols for cardiopulmonary emergencies and other internal and external disasters such as fire.
- The facility should have medications, equipment, and written protocols available to treat malignant hyperthermia when triggering agents are used.
- The facility should have a written protocol in place for the safe and timely transfer of patients to a prespecified alternate care facility when extended or emergency services are needed to protect the health or well-being of the patient.

Appendix 2

AMERICAN SOCIETY OF ANESTHESIOLOGISTS' STATEMENT ON SAFE USE OF PROPOFOL (APPROVED BY ASA HOUSE OF DELEGATES ON OCTOBER 27, 2004)

Because sedation is a continuum, it is not always possible to predict how an individual patient will respond. Owing to the potential for rapid, profound changes in sedative/anesthetic depth and the lack of antagonist medications, agents such as propofol require special attention. Even if moderate sedation is intended, patients receiving propofol should receive care consistent with that required for deep sedation.

The American Society of Anesthesiologists (ASA) believes that the involvement of an anesthesiologist in the care of every patient undergoing anesthesia is optimal. However, when this is not possible, nonanesthesia personnel who administer propofol should be qualified to rescue[1] patients whose level of sedation becomes deeper than initially intended and who enter, if briefly, a state of general anesthesia.[2]

The physician responsible for the use of sedation/anesthesia should have the education and training to manage the potential medical complications of sedation/anesthesia. The physician should be proficient in airway management, have advanced life support skills appropriate for the patient population, and understand the pharmacology of the drugs used.

The physician should be physically present throughout the sedation and remain immediately available until the patient is medically discharged from the postprocedure recovery area.

The practitioner administering propofol for sedation/anesthesia should, at a minimum, have the education and training to identify and manage the airway and cardiovascular changes which occur in a patient who enters a state of general anesthesia, as well as the ability to assist in the management of complications.

The practitioner monitoring the patient should be present throughout the procedure and be completely dedicated to that task.

During the administration of propofol, patients should be monitored without interruption to assess level of consciousness, and to identify early signs of hypotension, bradycardia, apnea, airway obstruction and/or oxygen desaturation. Ventilation, oxygen saturation, heart rate (HR), and blood pressure (BP) should be monitored at regular and frequent intervals. Monitoring for the presence of exhaled carbon dioxide should be utilized when possible, because movement of the chest will not dependably identify airway obstruction or apnea.

Age-appropriate equipment must be immediately available for the maintenance of a patent airway, oxygen enrichment, and artificial ventilation in addition to circulatory equipment.

[1] Rescue of a patient from a deeper level of sedation than intended is an intervention by a practitioner proficient in airway management and advanced life support. The qualified practitioner corrects adverse physiologic consequences of the deeper-than-intended level of sedation (such as hypoventilation, hypoxia, and hypotension) and returns the patient to the originally intended level. It is not appropriate to continue the procedure at an unintended level of sedation.

[2] The statement in the American Association of Nurse Anesthetists (AANA)–ASA Joint Statement regarding Propofol Administration, dated April 14, 2004, that reads, "Whenever propofol is used for sedation/anesthesia, it should be administered only by persons trained in the administration of general anesthesia, who are not simultaneously involved in these surgical or diagnostic procedures. This restriction is concordant with specific language in the propofol package insert, and failure to follow these recommendations could put patients at increased risk of significant injury or death," is consistent with the principles set forth in this statement.

In addition, some states have prescriptive regulations concerning the administration of propofol. There are different considerations when propofol is given to intubated, ventilated patients in a critical care setting.

Similar concerns apply when other intravenous induction agents are used for sedation, such as thiopental, methohexital, or etomidate. Administering combinations of drugs including sedatives and analgesics may increase the likelihood of adverse outcomes.

For additional information on the continuum of sedation and on sedation by nonanesthesiologists, we refer you to the ASA's documents "Continuum of Depth of Sedation: Definition of General Anesthesia and Levels of Sedation/ Analgesia" and "Practice Guidelines for Sedation and Analgesia by Non-Anesthesiologists." ASA's documents that address additional perioperative care issues are the "Guidelines for Office-Based Anesthesia," "Guidelines for Ambulatory Anesthesia and Surgery" and "Practice Guidelines for Preoperative Fasting and the Use of Pharmacologic Agents to Reduce the Risk of Pulmonary Aspiration."

All ASA documents can be found on the website, www.ASAhq.org

The Warnings section of the drug's package insert (Diprivan, AstraZeneca 4-01, accessed 7-04) states that propofol used for sedation or anesthesia "should be administered only by persons trained in the administration of general anesthesia and not involved in the conduct of the surgical/diagnostic procedure."

Appendix 3

STATEMENT ON THE LABELING OF PHARMACEUTICALS FOR USE IN ANESTHESIOLOGY (APPROVED BY ASA HOUSE OF DELEGATES ON OCTOBER 27, 2004)

Rationale:

The practice of anesthesiology requires the administration of a wide variety of potent medications. These medications are often given in high acuity situations and in environments with poor visibility and multiple distractions. Medications with widely differing actions, such as muscle relaxants, vasopressors, and vasodilators, are often used in the course of a single anesthetic, at times simultaneously. It has been recognized for some time that perioperative medication errors are a significant potential source of morbidity and, rarely, mortality. Interest in medication errors has extended to regulatory agencies, the federal government, and the general public.

The recognition and identification of an object depends on shape, color, brightness, and contrast. As these elements become increasingly distinctive, identification of the object becomes faster and more accurate. Therefore, although multiple factors contribute to medication errors, consistency and clarity of pharmaceutical and syringe labeling, in accordance with human factors, are important elements in their prevention.

Statement:

The primary consideration in the design of labels for pharmaceutical containers should be patient safety and the reduction of medication errors. This is particularly true for the potent medications used in the practice of anesthesiology. Therefore, the American Society of Anesthesiologists (ASA) supports the manufacture and use of pharmaceuticals with labels meeting the following standards, which are consistent with those established by the American Society for Testing and Materials International (ASTM International):

1. *Label content:* The drug's generic name, concentration, and volume or total contents of the vial or ampoule should be the most prominent items displayed on the label of each vial or ampoule containing pharmaceuticals for use in the practice of anesthesiology. In addition, the drug's proprietary name, manufacturer, lot number, date of manufacture, and expiration date should also be included on the label.
2. *Font:* The text on the label should be designed to enhance the recognition of the drug name and concentration as recommended in ASTM International standards D4267, Standard Specification for Labels for Small-Volume Parenteral Drug Containers and D6398, Standard Practice to Enhance Identification of Drug Names on Labels (Section 7). These standards include recommendations for the font size, extra space for separation around the drug name, and the use of additional emphasis for the initial syllable, or a distinctive syllable, of similar drug names.
3. *Contrasting background:* Maximum contrast between the text and background should be provided by high-contrast color combinations, as specified in Section 6.3.1 of ASTM International Standard D6398, which also minimize the impact of color blindness:

Text	Background
Black	White
Blue	Yellow
White	Blue
Blue	White

4. *Color:* Nine classes of drugs commonly used in the practice of anesthesiology have a standard background color established for user-applied syringe labels by ASTM International Standard D4774, Standard Specifications for User Applied Drug Labels in Anesthesiology. For these drugs, the color of the container's top, label border, and any other colored area on the label, excluding the background as required for maximum contrast, should be the color corresponding to the drug's classification.

The color would be that established in Standard D4774 and therefore identical to the color of the corresponding syringe label.

Drug Class	Pantone Color
Induction agents	Yellow
Tranquilizers	Orange 151
Muscle relaxants	Fluorescent red 805
Relaxant antagonists	Fluorescent red 805/white diagonal stripes
Narcotics	Blue 297
Narcotic antagonists	Blue 297/white diagonal stripes
Major tranquilizers	Salmon 156
Narcotic/tranquilizer combinations	Blue 297/salmon 156
Vasopressors	Violet 256
Hypotensive agents	Violet 256/white diagonal stripes
Local anesthetics	Gray 401
Anticholinergic agents	Green 367

5. *Bar coding:* Essential information including the drug's generic name, concentration, and volume of the vial or ampoule should be bar coded at a location on the vial or ampoule which will not interfere with the label's legibility, as specified in ASTM International Standard D6398 Section 8.

Appendix 4

AMERICAN SOCIETY OF ANESTHESIOLOGISTS' DEFINITIONS OF MONITORED ANESTHESIA CARE

As with all American Society of Anesthesiologists (ASA) official statements and guidelines, ASA's *Position on Monitored Anesthesia Care* came due for a periodic review. With the Committee on Economics input, several substantive changes to the statement were made in 2003. Because the revised position statement significantly alters the definition of monitored anesthesia care (MAC), ASA members need to understand the reasons for, and implications of these changes.

History of Monitored Anesthesia Care

Until the mid-1980s, anesthesiologists classified anesthesia into three types: general, regional, and local standby. The Tax Equity and Fiscal Responsibility Act (TEFRA) of 1982 acknowledged that "standby anesthesia" was a physician service and therefore payable under Medicare Part B. Consequently the Health Care Financing Administration (now the Centers for Medicare & Medicaid Services) amended the Medicare Carrier Manual to tell the carriers to pay for standby anesthesia "...the same as for any other anesthesia procedure." Taken together, TEFRA and the Medicare Carrier Manual supported standby anesthesia as a full service subject to an unreduced payment.

Some payers did not interpret "standby" the same way that Medicare did. To eliminate confusion about the standby issue, ASA replaced "standby anesthesia" with "monitored anesthesia care." The House of Delegates approved the first position statement on MAC in 1986. By dropping the baggage attached to "standby anesthesia," ASA intended the new term to demonstrate that the anesthesiologist was actively involved in patient care. The 1986 position statement read, in part:

The phrase "Monitored Anesthesia Care" refers to instances in which an anesthesiologist has been called upon to provide specific anesthesia services to a particular patient undergoing a planned procedure, in connection with which a patient receives local anesthesia, or in some cases, no anesthesia at all. In such a case, the anesthesiologist is providing specific services to the patient and is in control of the patient's nonsurgical or nonobstetrical medical care, including the responsibility of monitoring of the patient's vital signs, and is available to administer anesthetics or provide other medical care as appropriate.

In 1998, then-ASA president William D. Owens, referred the MAC statement to both the Committee on Economics and the Committee on Surgical Anesthesia for review. After lengthy and spirited discussions, a revised statement was presented to the 1998 House of Delegates and was adopted. The 1998 statement reaffirmed that "MAC is a specific anesthesia service in which an anesthesiologist has been requested to participate in the care of a patient undergoing a diagnostic or therapeutic procedure."

The 1998 version also stated that:

Monitored anesthesia care often includes the administration of doses of medications for which the loss of normal protective reflexes or loss of consciousness is likely. Monitored anesthesia care refers to those situations in which the patient remains able to protect the airway for the majority of the procedure. If, for an extended period of time, the patient is rendered unconscious and/or loses protective reflexes, then anesthesia care shall be considered a general anesthetic.

Shortly before the 1998 revision, the concept of a sedation continuum became part of ASA's efforts to educate nonanesthesiologists about conscious sedation. Changes to the 1998 MAC statement highlight the concept of the sedation continuum to illustrate the overlap between conscious sedation, MAC, and general anesthesia.

Position Statement

Although the 1998 MAC statement effectively addressed a number of thorny issues, many ASA members thought the expressions "extended period" and "majority of the procedure" were vague and seemed to indicate that an anesthetic was an MAC unless the patient was unconscious for >50% of the procedure. With the increasing use of propofol and similar agents for sedation, sometimes lightheartedly referred to as a *Big MAC*, the dividing line between general anesthesia and MAC became increasingly blurred, highlighting the need for further refinement of the MAC statement.

In 2003 the Committee on Economics proposed major changes to the statement. These changes included both a revision and expansion of the services that may be provided during MAC, a statement affirming equal payment for MAC compared with other anesthesia services and a clear dividing line between MAC and general anesthesia. The committee addressed the last issue by including the following text:

If the patient loses consciousness and the ability to respond purposefully, the anesthesia care is a general anesthetic, irrespective of whether airway instrumentation is required.

Increasing Prevalence of Monitored Anesthesia Care Payment Policies

While the committee struggled with a better definition of MAC, many payers were addressing when MAC is medically necessary. From the perspective of Medicare and other health insurers, the request of a physician or patient alone is not sufficient to justify payment for anesthesia care for a particular procedure. By law, the Medicare program forbids payment for services unless those services are medically necessary. Although Medicare has never published a national policy on MAC and medical necessity, many Medicare carriers have done so.

In considering when MAC is medically necessary, many Medicare carriers have determined that certain diagnostic and therapeutic procedures do not "usually" require the services of an anesthesiologist. These services include procedures where conscious sedation is "inherent" (and therefore not separately payable). They also include many minor or minimally invasive diagnostic or therapeutic procedures where sedation or anesthesia is rarely needed. Carriers may adopt and publish Local Coverage Determinations (LCDs) to inform participating providers of the payment rules. A typical MAC LCD will include a list of services where MAC is deemed unnecessary without meeting medical necessity requirements, which are often defined through a long list of ICD-9 diagnosis codes. The model MAC policy adopted by some carriers and rejected by others in the mid-1990s provided the basis for this structure.

Anesthesiologists serving on carrier advisory committees or state anesthesiology societies and individual anesthesiologists have taken active roles in working with Medicare carriers during development of MAC policies. Frequently, the carrier has substantially altered the proposed MAC LCD to address the legitimate concerns of these participants.

Medicare introduced the "QS" modifier in 1992 for reporting MAC services. Several private payers require reporting the QS to track the use of MAC. With the recent change in the definition of MAC, the reporting frequency for QS will likely decrease, and the Committee on Economics will closely follow the response of health insurers to this anticipated change.

Threats Going Forward

Worker shortages involving anesthesia delivery combined with increasing numbers of procedures performed under sedation have led some nonanesthesiologist physicians to provide sedation services for other physicians. Those who provide these second-physician conscious sedation services are discovering obstacles involving payment. The current conscious sedation codes cannot be used because they only apply to the physician performing the operative procedure.

According to Current Procedural Terminology guidelines, the second physician is instructed to use the anesthesia codes to report sedation services. Recognizing that anesthesia and conscious sedation services differ significantly, most private payers refuse to pay for the conscious sedation second-physician service when billed as anesthesia. The pressure from the rest of organized medicine to establish a method for nonanesthesiologists to report and bill for sedation is rising rapidly.

Conscious sedation and the newly revised MAC service appear superficially similar, and the terms are too often used interchangeably. Our specialty faces the risk that payers may reduce MAC payments to the much lower conscious sedation levels. The Committee on Economics intends to present a clear and compelling case that MAC and conscious sedation are fundamentally different services, justifying payments for MAC at the same level as for other anesthetic techniques.

Conclusions

ASA's MAC statement has been substantially revised this past year, providing improved guidance on the differences between MAC and general anesthesia. This improved definition will lead to significant reductions in the number of anesthetics reported as MAC and subject to the many MAC payment policies in the public and private sector. Nonanesthesiologists providing conscious sedation services are lobbying aggressively for a method to receive recognition for their work; however, this recognition may create a downward pressure on the value assigned for MAC services, an issue to which ASA remains attentive.

Anesthesiologists from a wide spectrum of practice styles represent the various interests and viewpoints of ASA as members of the Committee on Economics. The Committee on Economics strives to develop policies that are reasonable, rational, and appropriate for ASA as a whole. Individual members of ASA have access to the committee directly or through their state society's delegates to the ASA House of Delegates. The committee invites and welcomes input on economic issues that concern the practice of anesthesiology.

Appendix 5

ANESTHESIA APPARATUS CHECKOUT RECOMMENDATIONS, 1993

This checkout, or a reasonable equivalent, should be conducted before administration of anesthesia. These recommendations are only valid for an anesthesia system that conforms to current and relevant standards and includes an ascending bellows ventilator and at least the following monitors: capnograph, pulse oximeter, oxygen analyzer, respiratory volume monitor (spirometer) and breathing system pressure monitor with high and low pressure alarms. This is a guideline which users are encouraged to modify to accommodate differences in equipment design and variations in local clinical practice. Such local modifications should have appropriate peer review. Users should refer to the operator's manual for the manufacturer's specific procedures and precautions, especially the manufacturer's low-pressure leak test (step No. 5).

Emergency Ventilation Equipment
1. **Verify backup ventilation equipment is available and functioning**[1]

High Pressure System
1. **Check O_2 cylinder supply**[1]
   a. Open O_2 cylinder and verify at least half full (approximately 1,000 psi).
   b. Close cylinder.
2. **Check central pipeline supplies**[1]
   a. Check that hoses are connected and pipeline gauges read about 50 psi.

Low Pressure System
1. **Check initial status of low pressure system**[1]
   a. Close flow control valves and turn vaporizers off.
   b. Check fill level and tighten vaporizers' filler caps.
2. **Perform leak check of machine low pressure system**[1]
   a. Verify that the machine master switch and flow control valves are OFF.
   b. Attach "Suction Bulb" to common Fresh gas outlet.
   c. Squeeze bulb repeatedly until fully collapsed.
   d. Verify bulb stays *fully* collapsed for at least 10 seconds.
   e. Open one vaporizer at a time and repeat 'c' and 'd' as above.
   f. Remove suction bulb, and reconnect fresh gas hose.
3. **Turn on machine master switch**[1] and all other necessary electrical equipment.
4. **Test flowmeters**[1]
   a. Adjust flow of all gases through their full range, checking for smooth operation of floats and undamaged flow tubes.
   b. Attempt to create a hypoxic O_2/N_2O mixture and verify correct changes in flow and/or alarm.

Scavenging System
1. **Adjust and check scavenging system**[1]
   a. Ensure proper connections between the scavenging system and both APL (pop-off) valve and ventilator relief valve.
   b. Adjust waste gas vacuum (if possible).
   c. Fully open APL valve and occlude Y-piece.

---

[1]If an anesthesia provider uses the same machine in successive cases, these steps need not be repeated or may be abbreviated after the initial checkout.

d. With minimum O_2 flow, allow scavenger reservoir bag to collapse completely and verify that absorber pressure gauge reads approximately zero.

e. With the O_2 flush activated allow the scavenger reservoir bag to distend fully, and then verify that absorber pressure gauge reads <10 cm H_2O.

Breathing System

1. **Calibrate O_2 monitor[1]**
   a. Ensure monitor reads 21% in room air.
   b. Verify low O_2 alarm is enabled and functioning.
   c. Reinstall sensor in circuit and flush breathing system with O_2.
   d. Verify that monitor now reads >90%.

2. **Check initial status of breathing system**
   a. Set selector switch to "Bag" mode.
   b. Check that breathing circuit is complete, undamaged, and unobstructed.
   c. Verify that CO_2 absorbent is adequate.
   d. Install breathing circuit accessory equipment (e.g. humidifier, PEEP valve) to be used during the case.

3. **Perform leak check of the breathing system**
   a. Set all gas flows to zero (or minimum).
   b. Close APL (pop-off) valve and occlude Y-piece.
   c. Pressurize breathing system to approximately 30 cm H_2O with O_2 flush.
   d. Ensure that pressure remains fixed for at least 10 seconds.
   e. Open APL (pop-off) valve and ensure that pressure decreases.

Manual and Automatic Ventilation Systems

1. **Test ventilation systems and unidirectional valves**
   a. Place a second breathing bag on Y-piece.
   b. Set appropriate ventilator parameters for next patient.
   c. Switch to automatic ventilation (ventilator) mode.
   d. Fill bellows and breathing bag with O_2 flush and then turn ventilator ON.
   e. Set O_2 flow to minimum, other gas flows to zero.
   f. Verify that during inspiration bellows delivers appropriate tidal volume and that during expiration bellows fills completely.
   g. Set fresh gas flow to approximately 5 L/min.
   h. Verify that the ventilator bellows and simulated lungs fill and empty appropriately without sustained pressure at end expiration.
   i. Check for proper action of unidirectional valves.
   j. Exercise breathing circuit accessories to ensure proper function.
   k. Turn ventilator OFF and switch to manual ventilation (Bag/APL) mode.
   l. Ventilate manually and assure inflation and deflation of artificial lungs and appropriate feel of system resistance and compliance.
   m. Remove second breathing bag from Y-piece.

Monitors

1. **Check, calibrate and/or set alarm limits of all monitors**
   a. Capnometer
   b. Pulse oximeter
   c. Oxygen analyzer
   d. Respiratory volume monitor (Spirometer)
   e. Pressure monitor with high and low airway alarms

Final Position

1. **Check final status of machine**
   a. Vaporizers off
   b. APL valve open
   c. Selector switch to "Bag"
   d. All flowmeters to zero
   e. Patient suction level adequate
   f. Breathing system ready to use

Appendix 6

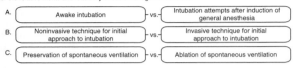

DIFFICULT AIRWAY ALGORITHM

1. Assess the likelihood and clinical impact of basic management problems:

    A. Difficult ventilation
    B. Difficult intubation
    C. Difficult with patient cooperation or consent
    D. Difficult tracheostomy

2. Actively pursue oppurtunities to deliver supplemental oxygen throughout the process of difficult airway management

3. Consider the relative merits and feasibility of basic management choices:

    A.   Awake intubation   vs.   Intubation attempts after induction of general anesthesia

    B.   Noninvasive technique for initial approach to intubation   vs.   Invasive technique for initial approach to intubation

    C.   Preservation of spontaneous ventilation   vs.   Ablation of spontaneous ventilation

4. Develop primary and alternative strategies:

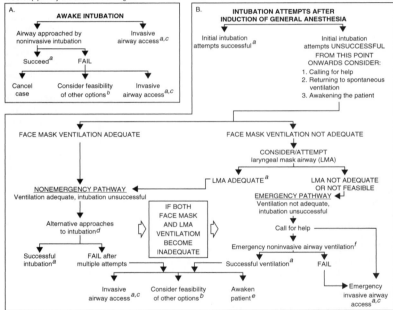

^{a} **Confirm ventilation, tracheal intubation, or LMA placement with exhaled CO_2**

^{b} Other options include (but are not limited to): surgery utilizing face mask or LMA anesthesia, local anesthesia infiltration or regional nerve blockade. Pursuit of these options usually implies that mask ventilation will not be problematic. Therefore, these options may be of limited value if this step in the algorithm has been reached through the Emergency Pathway.

^{c} Invasive airway access includes surgical or percutaneous tracheostomy or cricothyrotomy.

^{d} Alternative noninvasive approaches to difficult intubation include (but are not limited to): use of different laryngoscopes blades, LMA as an intubation conduit (with or without fiberoptic guidance), fiberoptic intubation, intubating stylet or tube changer, light wand, retrograde intubation, and blind oral or nasal intubation.

^{e} Consider repreparation of the patient for awake intubation or cancelling surgery.

^{f} Options for emergency noninvasive airway ventilation include (but are not limited to): rigid bronchoscope, esophageal–tracheal combitube ventilation, or transtracheal jet ventilation

Appendix 7

ADVANCED CARDIAC LIFE SUPPORT (ACLS) UPDATES, DECEMBER 2005 (FOR DETAILED ALGORITHMS REFER TO THE AMERICAN HEART ASSOCIATION GUIDELINES)

1. Performance of high quality cardiopulmonary resuscitation (CPR), including early CPR, defibrillation (for sudden witnessed collapse), airway maintenance, adequate rate, and depth of chest compressions with minimal interruptions. Chest compression/ventilation ratio of 30:2 (one or two rescuers) or 15:2 (two rescuers for infants and children only).

2. Increased use of laryngeal mask airways (LMAs) and endotracheal tubes by providers with adequate training. If an advanced airway is introduced, then chest compressions should be at the rate of 100 per minute with 8 to 10 breaths per minute.

3. Confirmation of proper endotracheal tube placement both by clinical assessment and using a device/detector.

4. Organization of care to minimize interruptions of chest compressions, breath delivery, or to gain vascular access. Chest compressors should change every 2 minutes.

5. Adequate administration of drugs, as soon as possible, during CPR after rhythm checks. Epinephrine may be given every 3 to 5 minutes. Vasopressin (one dose) may be given after the first or second shock (see subsequent text).

6. Pulseless arrest: uninterrupted CPR for 5 cycles per 2 minutes. CPR resumed immediately after delivery of one shock without pulse or rhythm check. All pulse or rhythm checks are performed after 5 cycles per 2 minutes.

7. Ventricular fibrillation/pulseless ventricular tachycardia: administration of amiodarone/lidocaine to be considered once—two to three shocks have already been delivered with adequate CPR and vasopressor administration.

8. Asystole: epinephrine 1 mg IV every 3 to 5 minutes, one dose of vasopressin (40 units IV), atropine 1 mg IV (up to 3 mg).

9. Symptomatic bradycardia: urgent preparation for transcutaneous pacing, atropine 0.5 mg IV (up to 3 mg), epinephrine or dopamine infusion (if atropine is ineffective).

10. Tachycardia: synchronized cardioversion for the unstable patient. For the stable patient, treatment should be initiated after a 12-lead electrocardiogram (ECG) to differentiate between narrow and wide complex tachycardia.

11. Adequate glucose control and even hypothermia may be induced for its neurocoronary protective effects.

Appendix 8

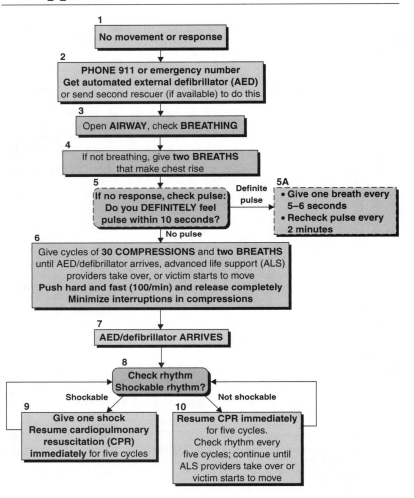

1 No movement or response

2 **PHONE 911 or emergency number**
   Get automated external defibrillator (AED)
   or send second rescuer (if available) to do this

3 Open **AIRWAY**, check **BREATHING**

4 If not breathing, give **two BREATHS**
   that make chest rise

5 **If no response, check pulse:**
   Do you DEFINITELY feel
   pulse within 10 seconds?

   Definite pulse →

5A • **Give one breath every**
   5–6 seconds
   • **Recheck pulse every**
   2 minutes

   No pulse

6 Give cycles of **30 COMPRESSIONS** and **two BREATHS**
   until AED/defibrillator arrives, advanced life support (ALS)
   providers take over, or victim starts to move
   Push hard and fast (100/min) and release completely
   Minimize interruptions in compressions

7 **AED/defibrillator ARRIVES**

8 **Check rhythm**
   Shockable rhythm?

   Shockable   Not shockable

9 **Give one shock**
   Resume cardiopulmonary
   resuscitation (CPR)
   immediately for five cycles

10 **Resume CPR immediately**
   for five cycles.
   Check rhythm every
   five cycles; continue until
   ALS providers take over or
   victim starts to move

Appendix 9

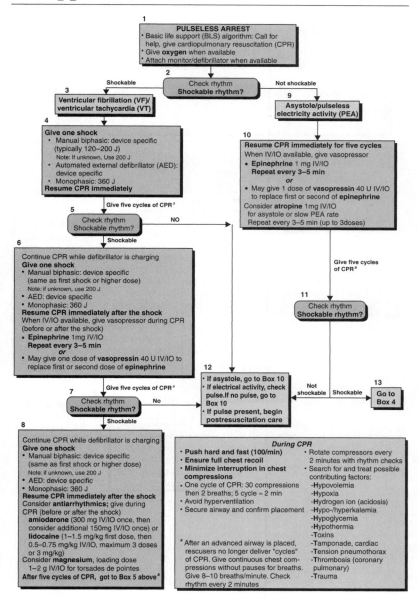

Appendix 10

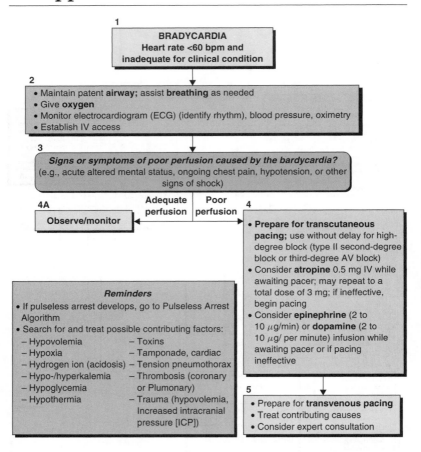

1

BRADYCARDIA
Heart rate <60 bpm and
inadequate for clinical condition

2
- Maintain patent **airway**; assist **breathing** as needed
- Give **oxygen**
- Monitor electrocardiogram (ECG) (identify rhythm), blood pressure, oximetry
- Establish IV access

3
Signs or symptoms of poor perfusion caused by the bardycardia?
(e.g., acute altered mental status, ongoing chest pain, hypotension, or other signs of shock)

Adequate perfusion | **Poor perfusion**

4A
Observe/monitor

4
- **Prepare for transcutaneous pacing;** use without delay for high-degree block (type II second-degree block or third-degree AV block)
- Consider **atropine** 0.5 mg IV while awaiting pacer; may repeat to a total dose of 3 mg; if ineffective, begin pacing
- Consider **epinephrine** (2 to 10 μg/min) or **dopamine** (2 to 10 μg/ per minute) infusion while awaiting pacer or if pacing ineffective

5
- Prepare for **transvenous pacing**
- Treat contributing causes
- Consider expert consultation

Reminders
- If pulseless arrest develops, go to Pulseless Arrest Algorithm
- Search for and treat possible contributing factors:
  - Hypovolemia
  - Hypoxia
  - Hydrogen ion (acidosis)
  - Hypo-/hyperkalemia
  - Hypoglycemia
  - Hypothermia
  - Toxins
  - Tamponade, cardiac
  - Tension pneumothorax
  - Thrombosis (coronary or Plumonary)
  - Trauma (hypovolemia, Increased intracranial pressure [ICP])

Appendix 11

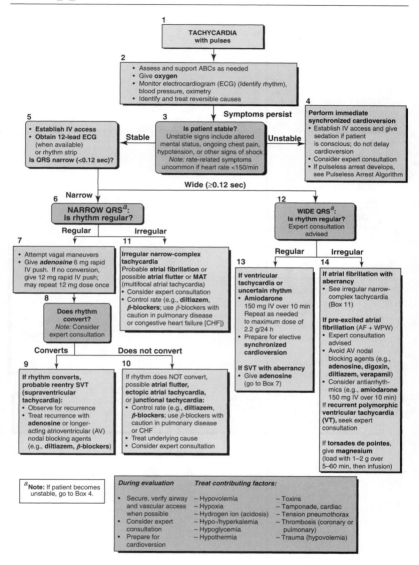

1
TACHYCARDIA
with pulses

2
- Assess and support ABCs as needed
- Give **oxygen**
- Monitor electrocardiogram (ECG) (Identify rhythm), blood pressure, oximetry
- Identify and treat reversible causes

Symptoms persist

4
Perform immediate synchronized cardioversion
- Establish IV access and give sedation if patient is conscious; do not delay cardioversion
- Consider expert consultation
- If pulseless arrest develops, see Pulseless Arrest Algorithm

5
- Establish IV access
- Obtain 12-lead ECG (when available) or rhythm strip

Is QRS narrow (<0.12 sec)?

Stable

3
Is patient stable?
Unstable signs include altered mental status, ongoing chest pain, hypotension, or other signs of shock
Note: rate-related symptoms uncommon if heart rate <150/min

Unstable

Narrow

Wide (≥0.12 sec)

6
NARROW QRS[a]:
Is rhythm regular?

Regular   Irregular

12
WIDE QRS[a]:
Is rhythm regular?
Expert consultation advised

Regular   Irregular

7
- Attempt vagal maneuvers
- Give **adenosine** 6 mg rapid IV push. If no conversion, give 12 mg rapid IV push; may repeat 12 mg dose once

11
Irregular narrow-complex tachycardia
Probable **atrial fibrillation** or possible **atrial flutter** or **MAT** (multifocal atrial tachycardia)
- Consider expert consultation
- Control rate (e.g., **diltiazem, β-blockers**; use β-blockers with caution in pulmonary disease or congestive heart failure [CHF]

8
Does rhythm convert?
Note: Consider expert consultation

Converts   Does not convert

9
If rhythm converts, probable reentry SVT (supraventricular tachycardia):
- Observe for recurrence
- Treat recurrence with **adenosine** or longer-acting atrioventricular (AV) nodal blocking agents (e.g., **diltiazem, β-blockers**)

10
If rhythm does NOT convert, possible **atrial flutter**, ectopic atrial tachycardia, or **junctional tachycardia:**
- Control rate (e.g., **diltiazem, β-blockers**; use β-blockers with caution in pulmonary disease or CHF
- Treat underlying cause
- Consider expert consultation

13
If ventricular tachycardia or uncertain rhythm
- **Amiodarone** 150 mg IV over 10 min Repeat as needed to maximum dose of 2.2 g/24 h
- Prepare for elective **synchronized cardioversion**

If SVT with aberrancy
- Give **adenosine** (go to Box 7)

14
If atrial fibrillation with aberrancy
- See irregular narrow-complex tachycardia (Box 11)

If pre-excited atrial fibrillation (AF + WPW)
- Expert consultation advised
- Avoid AV nodal blocking agents (e.g., **adenosine, digoxin, diltiazem, verapamil**)
- Consider antiarrhythmics (e.g., **amiodarone** 150 mg IV over 10 min)

If recurrent polymorphic ventricular tachycardia (VT), seek expert consultation

If **torsades de pointes**, give **magnesium** (load with 1–2 g over 5–60 min, then infusion)

[a]**Note:** If patient becomes unstable, go to Box 4.

During evaluation
- Secure, verify airway and vascular access when possible
- Consider expert consultation
- Prepare for cardioversion

Treat contributing factors:
- Hypovolemia
- Hypoxia
- Hydrogen ion (acidosis)
- Hypo-/hyperkalemia
- Hypoglycemia
- Hypothermia

- Toxins
- Tamponade, cardiac
- Tension pneumothorax
- Thrombosis (coronary or pulmonary)
- Trauma (hypovolemia)

Index